CW00903480

The Complete
English Cocker Spaniel

The Complete
English Cocker Spaniel

by
Connie Vanacore
and
Dale Hood

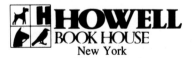

HOWELL
BOOK HOUSE
New York

COLLIER MACMILLAN CANADA
Toronto

MAXWELL MACMILLAN INTERNATIONAL
New York   Oxford   Singapore   Sydney

Howell Book House
Macmillan Publishing Company
866 Third Avenue, New York, NY 10022

Collier Macmillan Canada, Inc.
1200 Eglinton Avenue East, Suite 200
Don Mills, Ontario M3C 3N1

Library of Congress Cataloging-in-Publication Data
Vanacore, Connie.
    The complete English Cocker Spaniel / by Connie Vanacore and Dale Hood.
        p.   cm.
      ISBN 0-87605-117-4
      1. English cocker spaniel.   I. Hood, Dale.   II. Title.
    SF429.E47V36   1990
    636.7'52—dc20   89-26951   CIP

Macmillan books are available at special discounts for bulk purchases for sales promotions, premiums, fund-raising, or educational use. For details contact:

                            Special Sales Director
                            Macmillan Publishing Company
                            866 Third Avenue
                            New York, NY 10022

10 9 8 7 6 5 4 3 2 1

Printed in the United States of America

*This book is dedicated
to our devoted companions:*

Susan, Chip and Jason

Contents

About the Authors

CONNIE VANACORE has been a professional writer and editor for over twenty years. She was features editor of the American Kennel Club Gazette for eight years, and following that was the originator and editor of the veterinary column in that magazine for eight years.

She has owned Irish Setters for more than thirty-five years and has been active in specialty and all-breed clubs through most of that time.

She acquired her first English Cocker Spaniel—Ch. Fieldstone Black Eyed Susan (Ch. Maidavale Rosafe Citation ex Ch. Fieldstone Maesgywn Katrina)—from Fieldstone Kennels in 1981. Susan finished quickly and was bred in 1985 to Ch. Maidavale Grand Marnier to produce the black and white dog who is resident with his mother at the Vanacore house. He is Ch. Ballycroy Fieldstone Chip.

Connie is currently a free-lance writer, and is the author of *The New Complete Irish Setter*, co-authored with the late E. I. Eldredge.

DALE HOOD acquired her first English Cocker—Fieldstone Blue Velvet (Ch. Graecroft Starduster ex Lufnase Blue Becomes Me)—from Mary Ann Alston's Fieldstone Kennels in 1976. In 1980 the current English Cocker resident, an orange roan dog, came to Dale from Mary Ann. He is Ch. Foxfyre Fieldstone Phoenix (Ch. Trupence Fife and Drum ex Foxfyres Shady Lady).

Dale first became involved in the dog fancy in 1970, when she was active in obedience with her first Irish Setter. Shortly thereafter she purchased Ch. Foxfyre Scarlet Ember, CD, and became thoroughly immersed in the world of dogs.

Dale is active in all-breed and specialty clubs. She has been a member of the English Cocker Spaniel Club of America since 1978.

Preface

THIS BOOK is born out of love . . . a love of the English Cocker Spaniel as a breed, love of the individual dogs who have touched our lives and of the people who have been associated with and cherished these dogs as special.

The English Cocker Spaniel is a unique mixture of companion, sporting dog and show dog. A busy presence, with tail wagging and nose sniffing into every nook and cranny, belies a sweet and accommodating nature. The English Cocker is a friend, always ready for new adventure or perfectly content to sit beside you on the sofa, head on your knee as you read or watch television.

When properly conditioned and cared for, the English Cocker is a tireless hunter in the field. His compact body, hard pads and dense coat are well suited for work in water and on land, and he is probably the most underutilized hunting dog in the field today.

As a show dog his striking colors attract attention, and when he is on his toes he makes a worthy competitor for any of the larger sporting breeds. His gentle nature, however, sometimes conflicts with the demands of exaggerated motion. He would rather be at home, playing with his family, than out on the circuit. Overall, the latter is a more desirable trait for a companion, a quality in which the English Cocker excels.

The English Cocker is not a guard dog, although he certainly heralds the arrival of newcomers with a loud chorus. He could not be depended upon to defend the family homestead, though he would do his best to send out the word that some stranger is on the premises. He can be generous and demanding, boisterous and quiet all within a period of a few moments.

He wants to be with his people, does not suffer separation gladly and is most content in his home with his family around him, children most particularly. Being a childlike dog all his life, the English Cocker seems to have special affinity for children. They, in turn, respond to those long ears and soulful eyes as kindred spirits.

In this book we hope to portray the character of the English Cocker Spaniel, and to give those new to the breed some help in understanding and caring for this most special dog.

1

Evolution of the English Cocker Spaniel

The authors are indebted to Beth McKinney and Kate Romanski for use of material and photographs from The English Cocker Spaniel Jubilee Book *of the English Cocker Spaniel Club of America, Inc., published in 1986, to write this chapter.*

THE ENGLISH COCKER SPANIEL as we know it today is the result of the intermingling of several ancient breeds, all known under the general category of "spaniels."

"Spanyels" were thought to originate in Spain, according to references found in history books of the late 1300s, from hunting dogs of a long, low stature used for finding and flushing game. Paintings of the fourteenth and fifteenth centuries show spaniels of various colors both on the Continent and in England. Spanish dogs were particolored, often red and white or pied. There was also a strain of black and tan spaniels. In France at the same time a line of spaniels was developed with a mottled color, and these when bred with the partis gave rise to the roan patterns that we see today.

In England about the same time, spaniels were divided into classifications by size, weight and function. There were land spaniels and water spaniels. Water spaniels included the English Water Spaniel, now defunct as a breed, and the Irish Water Spaniel. Land spaniels included the Springer, the Sussex, the Clumber and the Field. Breeders were not averse to combining one with the other to achieve dogs that were useful for hunting various types of birds.

By the 1800s spaniels throughout Europe were evolving into two distinct types, the English-bred springing spaniel, which was primarily liver and white speckled, and the smaller, more diverse in color, cocking spaniel. The latter was used for hunting woodcock, hence the name, which has been associated with Cocker Spaniels ever since.

In the early days of dog shows in England, Field Spaniels were divided by weight, over twenty-five pounds and under twenty-five pounds; Cockers were in the latter category. In 1892 the Kennel Club gave the Cocker Spaniel separate identity in the Stud Book, and in 1901 the Spaniel Club in England abolished the weight limit for Cocker Spaniels. As a result, sturdy dogs with shorter backs and longer legs began to appear. In 1902 the Cocker Spaniel Club was formed.

It is interesting to note that the Cocker Spaniel as it is known worldwide is the English variety, which began to be imported to the United States in the late 1880s but evolved here as the American Cocker. Both English and American Cockers in the United States are descended from English Champion Obo.

OBO

All modern Cocker Spaniels, no matter what their country of registry, can be traced to a black, under-twenty-five-pound Field/Cocker Spaniel, Eng. Ch. Obo, bred by James Farrow of Ipswich, England, whelped June 14, 1879.

Obo enjoyed great success in England as a sire, establishing a line of long, low Cockers who were small and hardy enough to find game in low brush. In 1882 a breeder in New England, F. F. Pitcher, imported a black bitch, Chloe II, who was in whelp to Obo. In that litter was Obo II, the dog who is credited with founding the American Cocker Spaniel.

In England between 1880 and the early 1900s a different type of Cocker was being developed, a dog that eventually became the English Cocker Spaniel.

English breeders decided that the long, low dog personified by Obo was not the ideal hunter, so a dog was developed with more height at the shoulder and longer, stronger neck to retrieve game. Black

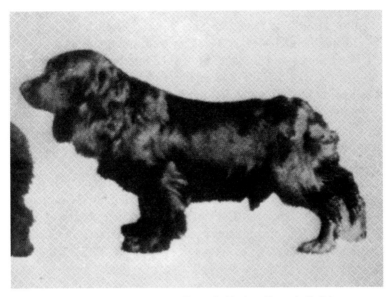

Eng. Ch. Obo, black dog (Farrow's Fred ex Farrow's Betty).

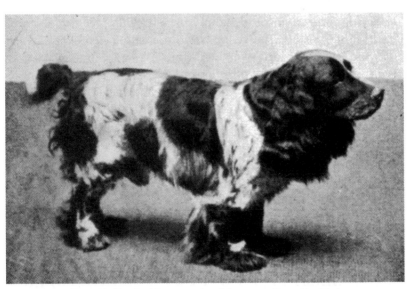

Braeside Bustle, blue roan dog (Viceroy ex Braeside Bizz).

3

remained the preferred color for many years, but roans and particolors began to be seen more frequently during this period. A blue roan dog named Braeside Bustle, whelped in 1894, is credited with being the progenitor of all blue roan and other colored English Cockers.

During the early 1900s, Cockers were imported both ways from the United States and England and were interbred and shown in the same classes. World War I reduced the trade between the two countries, but following the "Great War" the populations of dogs in both countries increased and importations resumed.

Each country was developing its own type, and in each a prepotent dog appeared that changed the course of both the American and English Cocker.

In the United States, on June 8, 1921, Red Brucie was whelped. This remarkable dog was bred by Herman Mellenthin, probably the most influential American Cocker breeder for the next twenty years. Red Brucie and his descendants established the American Cocker type as we know it today.

"OF WARE"

In 1875 in England, Mr. Richard Lloyd founded the "of Ware" Cockers. It was this line, including Ch. Obo, that produced the great dog Braeside Bustle. The kennel was eventually taken over by Richard's son, Herbert Lloyd, who bred countless litters for the next fifty-seven years and produced many record-making dogs in all colors.

The most famous dog acquired by that kennel, and the one who is behind all particolor and most solid-color English Cockers today, is English Ch. Invader of Ware. He was a dominant dog who was undefeated in the show ring, completed his championship by the time he was two years old and was a superior hunter, as well.

Herbert Lloyd brought some good-quality American solids to England to improve the lines there, and he also purchased an English-bred black, Bazel Otto, whelped in 1929, who became the dominant sire behind modern solid colors.

THE ENGLISH-TYPE COCKER COMES TO AMERICA

During World War I and until the early 1930s, English Cockers were rarely seen in the show ring in the United States. Some Canadian English Cockers, several of the "of Ware" suffix, worked their way

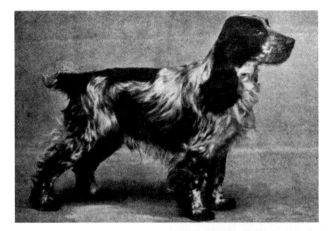

Ch. Invader of Ware, blue roan dog (Drumreaney Gunner ex Drumreaney Wonder).

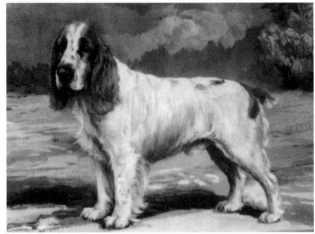

Ch. Blackmoor Beacon of Giralda, lemon and white dog (Blackmoor Brutus ex Blackmoor Bunting).

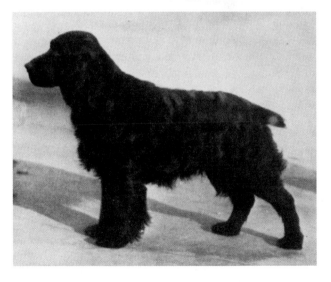

Bazel Otto, black dog (Joker of Padson ex Dunford Judy).

5

into American pedigrees, but it was not until 1932 and the importation of Mariner of Ware; a blue roan, Sterling of Ware; and a bitch, Lucky Maid of Ware, that the English Cocker began to make its mark.

Mariner was imported and owned by Atilla Cox of Louisville, Kentucky, and subsequently by Sydney Bufkin of Hazelhurst, Mississippi, where he was extensively used at stud.

Sterling of Ware was imported and owned by Priscilla St. George (Ryan) of Prune's Own Kennels, Tuxedo, New York, and he was bred to Mrs. W. K. DuPont's bitch, Lucky Maid, in 1933, to produce one of the breed's early champions, Ch. Squirrel Run Invasion.

In 1936, Geraldine Rockefeller Dodge (Mrs. M. Hartley Dodge), owner of Giralda Kennels, brought a lemon and white Cocker from England, Blackmoor Beacon of Giralda. Beacon was shown sparingly and was the first Group-placing English Cocker within the forty-eight states. He was more important as a sire, producing thirteen champions, and is behind most modern American-bred English Cockers.

Up until this time English-bred and American-bred Cockers were shown in the same classes, but in October 1935 the Cocker Spaniel Club of West Chester, Pennsylvania, held the first sanctioned Specialty show for English Cocker Spaniels in the United States. Following this, and with the help of English Cocker fancier Russell H. Johnson, Jr., who was the president of the American Kennel Club at the time, the AKC Board of Directors added English Cocker Spaniels to the list of varieties of distinct breeds eligible to be shown for championship competition. Following that decision in 1936, there were three varieties of Cocker: solid, particolor and English type. There was a Winners Dog and Winners Bitch in each variety, and then all three Best of Winners competed with any Specials for one Best of Breed. This system continued until 1942, when English Cockers were able to compete separately as a variety for Best of Breed and appeared in the Group.

All through the 1930s English-type and American Cockers continued to be interbred and competed in the show ring only for Best of Breed. Since there were fewer English-type Cockers, it was easier to win points in that variety, and many American Cockers won their titles by competing in the English variety classes.

2

English Cocker Spaniel Clubs and Breed Recognition

THE ENGLISH COCKER SPANIEL CLUB of America (ECSCA) is the Parent club for all organized English Cocker Spaniel activities in the United States. It is a member club of the American Kennel Club, to which it sends a Delegate, and it organizes shows and hunting trials for English Cockers. It also is the approving club for all local English Cocker club activities. It publishes a membership directory and a quarterly newsletter, which is sent to all members, and it is the guardian of the English Cocker Standard and the focal point for dissemination of all information pertaining to English Cocker health and welfare.

The English Cocker Spaniel Club was organized on June 20, 1936, at a meeting held at the home of Mr. and Mrs. E. Shippen Willing near Bryn Mawr, Pennsylvania. Mr. Willing was elected president of the club, a constitution and bylaws was adopted and other officers were elected. Twenty-six people became charter members at that meeting.

Eight months later, in February 1937, the first annual meeting was held. Membership, by invitation only, had grown to fifty-five.

The club held its first Specialty show on May 29, 1937, at Giralda Farms, where they continued to hold their Specialties for many years.

On October 28, 1938, at Giralda Farms, the fateful meeting was held in which it was resolved to cease interbreeding American and English-type Cocker Spaniels. In addition, the resolution opposed the showing of American Cockers in the English Cocker classes. The resolution defined an English Cocker to be a "dog or bitch of the Cocker Spaniel breed whose pedigree can be traced in all lines to dogs or bitches which were registered with the English Kennel Club (or eligible export pedigree) on or before January 1, 1930."

Although the goal of attaining separate breed status is implied in the resolution passed in 1938, it was not until 1946 that the American Kennel Club recognized the English Cocker Spaniel as a breed. Recognition came about largely because of the monumental pedigree research done by Geraldine Rockefeller Dodge, then president of the English Cocker Spaniel Club, and her curator of art, Josephine Z. Rine. English Cocker Spaniels appeared in the American Kennel Club Stud Book beginning in January 1947.

English Cockers had been judged under the English Standard, which was developed in the early 1900s. Once the decision had been made to separate the American from the English Cockers, the club formed a committee, under the advice of the American Kennel Club, to revise its Standard. This was accomplished in January 1945, after many months of discussion, and paved the way for the American Kennel Club to recognize the English Cocker Spaniel as a separate breed. The Standard has remained essentially the same, although it was slightly revised in 1955 and again in 1988.

ECSCA Specialty shows were suspended during World War II, but resumed in June 1947, with a show held in conjunction with the Bryn Mawr Kennel Club.

In 1948 a regional club was formed that called itself the English Cocker Spaniel Club of Northern California, with about twenty-six members. It lasted until 1959, when it was dissolved. During the 1950s and 1960s several other regional clubs were organized. The Twin Cities English Cocker Spaniel Club in Minnesota was formed in 1959 and lasted until 1969. The Heart of Michigan English Cocker Spaniel Club was also formed in 1959, but has flourished through the years.

It was not until 1975 that the next regional club was formed. The English Cocker Spaniel Club of Southern California was organized that year, followed by the Cascade English Cocker Spaniel Fanciers.

In 1977 the Parent club instituted a program to honor dogs working in the field. Working Certificates for Working Dog (WD) and Working Dog Excellent (WDX) were awarded for the first time that year. In 1978 obedience trials were added to the National Specialty for the first time.

Until 1979, with two exceptions when National Specialties were held in Ohio, all the annual fixtures were held on the East Coast. That year the National moved to Costa Mesa, California, to a record entry, including working tests, obedience, tracking and sweepstakes. Since that time, Nationals have rotated to different parts of the country, hosted usually by regional clubs, which have grown in number and importance.

In 1980 the English Cocker Spaniel Club of Northern California rose again. In Virginia and Maryland fanciers formed the Mason Dixon English Cocker Spaniel Club; the Seaboard English Cocker Spaniel Club is forming in the Carolinas; and in the Tampa area of Florida the Suncoast English Cocker Spaniel Club has organized. The North East English Cocker Spaniel Club is based in New England, and on the other coast the English Cocker Spaniel Club of San Diego came into being in 1979.

The growth of regional clubs dedicated to the breed is a reflection of the spread of the English Cocker throughout the country. Activity originally centered on the East Coast has spread within the past twenty years throughout the country. Midwest and West Coast breeders have come into their own, producing dogs of quality and type, integrating several lines into their breeding programs so that in most areas of the country today one can find English Cockers who are truly representative of the breed.

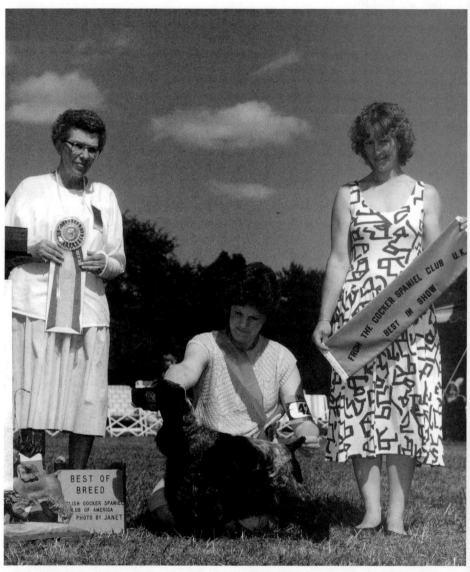

Ch. Olde Spice Sailors Beware, E.C.S.C.A. National Specialty Best of Breed winner, 1985 and 1986; breeder, owner and handler, Vicky Spice.

3

A Look at the English Cocker Spaniel Through Analysis of the Standard

---

THE ENGLISH COCKER is above all a dog that is pleasing to the eye. He comes as a neat package of moderate size, beautiful head, soft expression and friendly temperament wrapped in a coat of many and varied colors.

The Standard for any breed is the blueprint by which a breeder can measure the value of a dog in the show ring. No dog is perfect, but breeders strive, through careful study of the pedigrees and selection of the sire and dam, to come as close to the Standard as genetics allow.

The Standard for the English Cocker is quite comprehensive, and as we discuss it here, one should always keep in mind the total picture of an active, outgoing, sweet-natured dog.

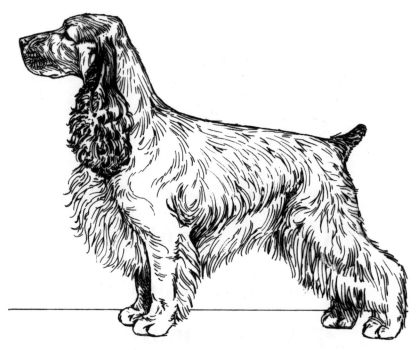

A correct English Cocker profile. *(All drawings in this chapter are by Pamela Powers.)*

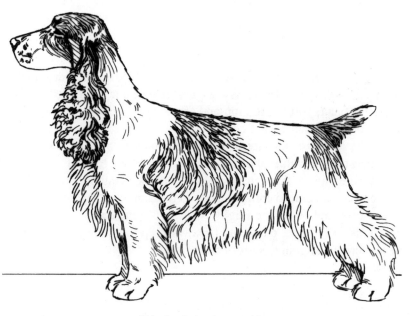

This dog is too long and low.

General Appearance

The English Cocker Spaniel is an active, merry sporting dog, standing well up at the withers and compactly built. He is alive with energy; his gait is powerful and frictionless, capable both of covering ground effortlessly and penetrating dense cover to flush and retrieve game. His enthusiasm in the field and the incessant action of his tail while at work indicate how much he enjoys the hunting for which he was bred. His head is especially characteristic. He is, above all, a dog of balance, both standing and moving, without exaggeration in any part, the whole worth more than the sum of its parts.

As we look at the English Cocker as a whole, we like to see a sturdy, upstanding, moderately sized dog, with a pleasing head and soft expression. It is a dog that looks all of a piece. Each part fits smoothly into the other so that there is no apparent break from neck to shoulder to loin to tail. A dog that is shelly, light boned, long or soft in back is incorrect. A dog that is in balance will have the angles of the shoulders and rear legs approximately the same. One does not want to see straight shoulders with hind legs stretched far out behind the dog. This leads to imbalance and an unsound dog.

Size, Proportion, Substance

Size—Height at withers: males 16 to 17 inches; females 15 to 16 inches. Deviations to be penalized. The most desirable weights—males 28 to 34 pounds; females 26 to 32 pounds. Proper conformation and substance should be considered more important than weight alone.

An English Cocker is not a smaller version of the English Springer Spaniel. It has its own characteristics of head and body type. It is shorter in back and cobbier than the Welsh Springer, while being somewhat smaller, and it is more refined in head and general appearance than its closest relative, the American Cocker.

An English Cocker that is smaller than the desired height tends to be dumpy or too light and unsubstantial in body. A dog that is taller than seventeen inches for males, sixteen inches for females, will either be too high on leg or, more likely, too big all over to retain the cobby, neat appearance that is desired.

It is difficult to assess the weight by looking at the dog in the ring, but usually a dog with proper bone and muscle will fall within the desired range. The exception is a dog that is too fat. A fat English Cocker (and because they love to eat, it is easy to have one that is overweight) will lack a waistline and will roll as it moves.

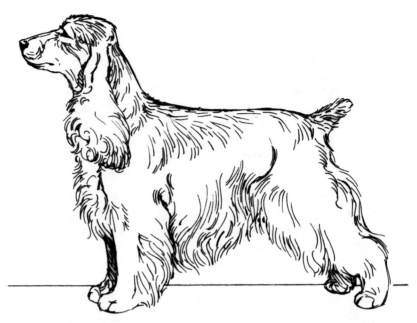

Snipey head, down-faced, with drop-off in back skull; neck does not blend smoothly into the shoulders.

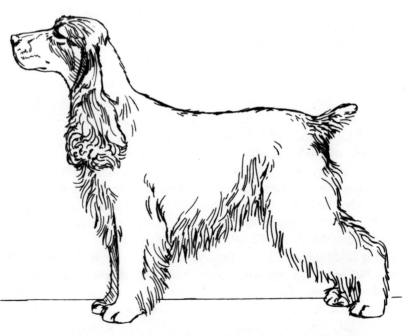

This dog is straight in the shoulder and his topline is soft and rumpy.

Proportion—Compactly built and short-coupled, with height at withers slightly greater than the distance from withers to set-on of tail.

Substance—The English Cocker is a solidly built dog with as much bone and substance as is possible without becoming cloddy or coarse.

A short-coupled dog means that the rib cage extends well back so there is not too much room between the end of the rib cage and the beginning of the thigh. Short-coupling gives the dog a compact, sturdy appearance, with no softness through the midsection. Bitches are sometimes slightly longer than males. The dog should be well up on leg and should never be long and low to the ground.

Head

General appearance—Strong, yet free from coarseness, softly contoured, without sharp angles. Taken as a whole, the parts combine to produce the expression distinctive of the breed.

The hallmark of the English Cocker is its head. It is moderately refined, with a soft, almost plushy look but with no excess flew or broad contours.

Expression—Soft, melting, yet dignified, alert, and intelligent.

The expression is most important and should be gentle, friendly, alert and soft.

Eyes—The eyes are essential to the desired expression. They are medium in size, full and slightly oval; set wide apart; lids tight. Haws are inconspicuous; may be pigmented or unpigmented. Eye color dark brown, except in livers and liver parti-colors where hazel is permitted, but the darker the hazel the better.

The eyes of the English Cocker convey the essence of the dog. They can be merry, sad, pleading, mischievous. They reflect the intelligence and sensitivity that are the hallmarks of the dog's temperament. Dark eyes are most desirable, the darker the better. Dark haws give a gentler, softer expression, even though the Standard does not require pigmented haws. White haws detract from the pleasing aspect of the face. Round eyes, light eyes and lack of pigment often create a startled or frightened expression, which is totally incorrect for the breed.

Ears—Set low, lying close to the head; leather fine, extending to the nose, well covered with long, silky, straight or slightly wavy hair.

English Cocker ears are long and set low. Feathering often extends to the shoulders and frames the face, adding to the soft expression.

Skull—Arched and slightly flattened when seen both from the side and from the front. Viewed in profile, the brow appears not appreciably higher than the back-skull. Viewed from above, the sides of the skull are in planes roughly parallel to those of the muzzle. Stop definite, but moderate, and slightly grooved.

Muzzle—Equal in length to skull; well cushioned; only as much narrower than the skull as is consistent with a full eye placement; cleanly chiselled under the eyes. Jaws strong, capable of carrying game. Nostrils wide for proper development of scenting ability; color black, except in livers and parti-colors of that shade where they will be brown; reds and parti-colors of that shade may be brown, but black is preferred. Lips square, but not pendulous or showing prominent flews.

Bite—Scissors. A level bite is not preferred. Overshot or undershot to be severely penalized.

The skull and muzzle should be about equal in length, with planes that are approximately parallel. Downfaced or snipey muzzles with lack of lip are incorrect. The stop should be evident, but one does not want to see a beetle-browed dog. The back skull should be equal in plane to the muzzle and should not drop off sharply to the rear. A dog with a dry mouth is preferred for delivering game, and a dog with strong jaws and teeth and without pendulous flews will not have a wet or slobbery mouth.

Neck, Topline and Body

Neck—Graceful and muscular, arched toward the head and blending cleanly, without throatiness, into sloping shoulders; moderate in length and in balance with the length and height of the dog.

The English Cocker's neck is of moderate length, strong without coarseness and held proudly. A swan neck, one that is too long and thin, or a ewe neck is incorrect. The neck must be muscular because the English Cocker when hunting is required to retrieve birds as big as ducks or pheasants.

Topline—The line of the neck blends into the shoulder and backline in a smooth curve. The backline slopes very slightly toward a gently rounded croup, and is free from sagging or rumpiness.

The topline is very important in furthering the impression of a cobby, strong, substantial dog. The neck and shoulder fit together

16

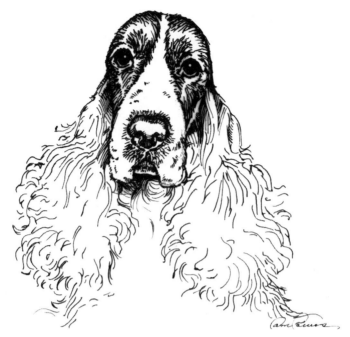

This is a correct English Cocker head.

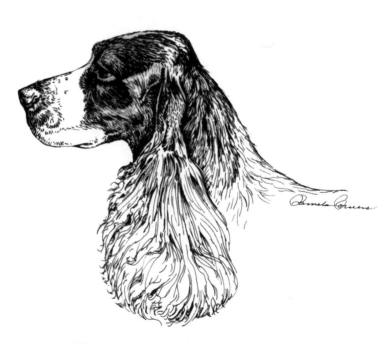

This is a correct English Cocker profile.

17

without noticeable break. Wide shoulders or withers that stick up above the level of the back are incorrect and spoil the smooth line from neck to tail. A topline that sags in the middle, or that falls off sharply with a steep slope, detracts from the square, sturdy appearance of the dog.

Body—Compact and well-knit, giving the impression of strength without heaviness. Chest deep; not so wide as to interfere with action of forelegs, nor so narrow as to allow the front to appear narrow or pinched. Forechest well developed, prosternum projecting moderately beyond shoulder points. Brisket reaches to the elbow and slopes gradually to a moderate tuck-up. Ribs well sprung and springing gradually to mid-body, tapering to back ribs which are of good depth and extend well back. Back short and strong. Loin short, broad and very slightly arched, but not enough to affect the topline appreciably. Croup gently rounded, without any tendency to fall away sharply.

The compact body is set foresquare on legs of ample bone. The front legs are well boned and straight, with no pinched-in appearance at the elbows or break at the ankles. The chest should come down as far as the elbows, and the underline of the body should be firm and muscular, with no sag to the stomach and only a moderate tuck-up under the loin.

Tail—Docked. Set on to conform to croup. Ideally, the tail is carried horizontally and is in constant motion while the dog is in action. Under excitement, the dog may carry his tail somewhat higher, but not cocked up.

The tail is docked to about one third its original length and should be carried straight out or slightly lifted to about two o'clock. A "terrier tail" is incorrect and spoils the outline of the dog.

Forequarters and Hindquarters

FOREQUARTERS

The English Cocker is moderately angulated. Shoulders are sloping, the blade flat and smoothly fitting. Shoulder blade and upper arm are approximately equal in length. Upper arm set well back, joining the shoulder with sufficient angulation to place the elbow beneath the highest point of the shoulder blade when the dog is standing naturally. Forelegs—Straight, with bone nearly uniform in size from elbow to heel; elbows set close to the body; pasterns nearly straight, with some flexibility. Feet—Proportionate in size to the legs, firm, round and catlike; toes arched and tight; pads thick.

18

Angulation moderate and, most importantly, in balance with that of the forequarters. Hips relatively broad and well rounded. Upper thighs broad, thick and muscular, providing plenty of propelling power. Second thighs well muscled and approximately equal in length to the upper. Stifle strong and well bent. Hock to pad short. Feet as in front.

The Standard stresses balance between forequarters and hindquarters. This means the dog should be all of a piece. The angles in the shoulders and upper arm match those of the hip, thighs and hocks. Moderation is the key word here. One does not want to see a straight shoulder or a long second thigh. The legs should be well boned and the feet should be round, with thick, close pads. Pointed or hare feet, feet that are flat or splayed, too big or spread are incorrect. The nails should be strong, usually black and kept short.

Coat

On head, short and fine; of medium length on body; flat or slightly wavy; silky in texture. The English Cocker is well-feathered, but not so profusely as to interfere with field work. Trimming is permitted to remove overabundant hair and to enhance the dog's true lines. It should be done so as to appear as natural as possible.

The coat should be silky and flat with sufficient feathering to be pleasing to the eye. An overabundance of coat is not desired, and dogs who do not carry profuse feathering should not be penalized. The coat should be shiny and healthy, with good texture which will vary according to color. Blacks and reds will tend to have a coat which is harder and denser to the touch without being coarse. The dark roans will have coat texture similar to the solids. Open-marked dogs with a predominance of white tend to have silkier coats with less abundant feathering.

The English Cocker is trimmed and hand stripped so that the top coat lies flat against the body. Some dogs are shown so tightly stripped and scissored that an unnatural appearance is created. Since the Standard calls for the coat to appear as natural as possible, excess trimming should be discouraged.

Color

Various. Parti-colors are either clearly marked, ticked or roaned, the white appearing in combination with black, liver or shades of red. In parti-colors it is preferable that solid markings be broken on the body and more or less evenly distributed; absence of body markings is acceptable. Solid colors are black, liver or shades of red. White feet on a solid are undesirable; a little white on throat is acceptable; but in neither case do these white markings make the dog a parti-color. Tan markings, clearly defined and of rich shade may appear in conjunction with black, livers and parti-color combinations of those colors. Black and tans and liver and tans are considered solid colors.

A group of English Cockers together is delightful in its diversity. Several colors can be found in a single litter of particolors. In the solid variety blacks, reds and black and tans can be found in the same litter. Generally, solids and partis are not interbred because of the possibility of mismarked puppies occurring in the litter. Although judges are supposed to be "color blind" when judging, some markings give illusions that are detrimental in the show ring. Even markings on the head and on the rear quarters, for instance, make a better impression than asymmetrical patches.

In solids marked with tan, symmetrical markings on the muzzle, above the eyes, on the neck, below the tail and on all four feet are desirable.

Gait

The English Cocker is capable of hunting in dense cover and upland terrain. His gait is accordingly characterized more by drive and the appearance of power than by great speed. He covers ground effortlessly and with extension both in front and rear, appropriate to his angulation. In the ring, he carries his head proudly and is able to keep much the same topline while in action as when standing for examination. Going and coming he moves in a straight line without crabbing or rolling, and with width between both front and rear legs appropriate to his build and gait.

The English Cocker is built with lots of heart and lung room and from puppyhood should be given room to run, play and hunt. With proper exercise and conditioning, this breed should be able to go all day with great vigor and stamina, and gait in the show ring should reflect this. This is not a racehorse, and should not be expected to keep up with an Irish Setter or a Pointer in stride, but the movement should be true and effortless. The English Cocker should look standing as in motion: balanced, with a firm topline, head up and with an alert expression full of interest and fun.

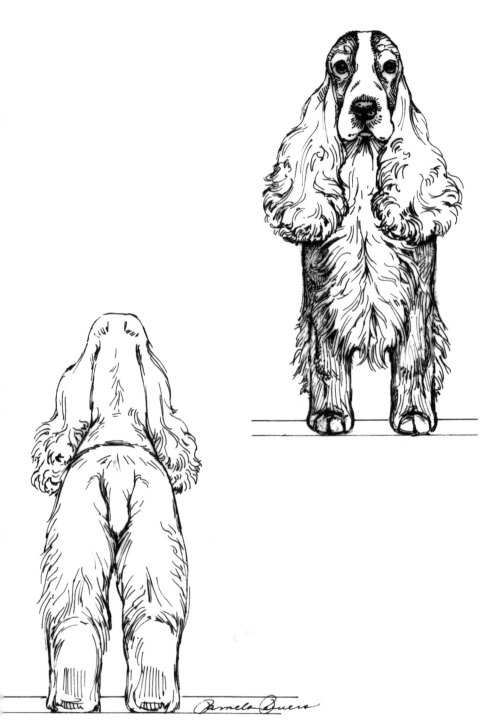

This shows a correct front and rear. Note the ample bone, well-developed thighs and sturdy appearance without coarseness.

Temperament

> The English Cocker is merry and affectionate, of equable disposition, neither sluggish nor hyperactive, a willing worker and a faithful and engaging companion.

The English Cocker is an ideal family dog, always friendly, willing to play or rest, energetic yet biddable. With proper socialization and exposure to people it makes a wonderful companion. One look at that wagging rear and soft expression is enough to melt the hardest heart.

JUDGING THE ENGLISH COCKER

The English Cocker is a difficult breed to judge. Those who are breeders first and judges later often look for qualities that those not intimately involved with the breed ignore.

"Type"—that elusive word which defines the essence of a breed—is more important to breeder-judges than to those less familiar with the breed. Type is found in the general appearance of the dog, in the head, expression and way of going. Breeder-judges will tend to forgive faults in movement or minor faults of construction if the dog has proper English Cocker type.

Sporting dog judges too often choose the dog with great reach and drive when seen gaiting from the side, when that is not the most important quality of the English Cocker. Often the dog with a long reach is one who is longer in body, compared to its height. According to the Standard, a long-bodied dog is incorrect. Too much emphasis is placed on side movement, to the detriment of viewing the dog as a whole.

Breeder-judges also realize that the temperament of the English Cocker is a soft one—that charging full tilt around the ring is not necessarily the hallmark of a good dog. Although the dog should be animated and show enjoyment and spirit, it need not be an out-of-control daredevil on a raceway. Judging should not be based on the dog who goes the fastest, but on the one whose movement shows power, stamina and control.

An English Cocker should be shown in hard condition, with plenty of muscle in the hindquarters. Judges should feel for that, because a dog who is soft cannot do a day's work in the field. Not to

22

be forgotten are the eye-pleasing qualities found in its distinctive head and expression and exquisite proportions throughout.

Moderation is the key to the English Cocker. Judges who keep that thought in mind will fault those dogs whose structure tends to the extreme. Before judging this breed, candidates should fix in their minds its important features, which are adequately expressed in the Standard.

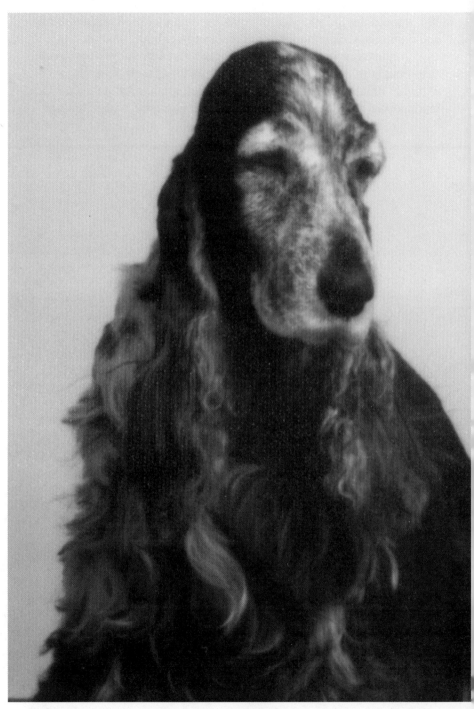

The English Cocker ages like fine wine: Ch. Canterbury's Elite at thirteen and a half years (Ch. Dunelm Galaxy ex Ch. Vari's Fascination).

4

Health and Care

THERE ARE NO SECRETS to raising a happy and healthy puppy. It does take time, attention and observation to give that puppy the best chance to grow into a sound, healthy adult.

If you have gone to a reputable breeder and purchased a puppy without obvious defects who has been well cared for, then you are on your way. Often the breeder will suggest, or insist, that you take your new puppy to your veterinarian for a checkup as soon as you get home.

This is a very good idea. It will assure you that you have a healthy dog and it will establish a relationship with a person who will play a big part in the life of your dog. To that first visit you should take a record from the breeder of the vaccinations the puppy has received. You should also take a stool sample, so the veterinarian can determine microscopically if your puppy is carrying internal parasites that would hinder proper growth. Many puppies do have worms, which are easily eliminated with appropriate medication.

If you live in a climate where heartworm disease is a problem, your veterinarian may want to take a small sample of blood to test for the presence of heartworms. If the test is negative, then you may want to start your puppy on preventative, a routine to be continued throughout a dog's life.

Once your puppy has been checked over and pronounced fit, then it is up to you to help growth and development, both mentally and physically, reach full genetic potential.

There are several excellent books, all about general dog care and training, that you can obtain in your bookstore or library, but there are things specific to the English Cocker that are important to know.

DIET

Your puppy should be fed a balanced ration three or four times a day. The breeder may have given you recommendations, and you should follow that diet until the puppy is well established in your home. Sudden changes will cause upsets to a puppy's sensitive system. There are many good commercial puppy and adult foods on the market. There is no need to supplement a good-quality brand-name food, and in fact the addition of some minerals, such as calcium, can have a detrimental effect on the normal growth patterns of the dog.

English Cockers tend to put on weight easily, so you will have to watch food intake to be sure your puppy does not get too fat. Puppies should be round and firm, but excess weight is not desirable.

HOUSE-TRAINING

English Cockers are sometimes not the easiest dogs to house-train. Patience and consistency are the keys. Be sure to use, but not abuse, a crate.

Crates, whether wire, wood, fiberglass or metal, are an indispensible part of a puppy's life. They provide a safe haven for the puppy to escape the activity of a household. They enable the puppy, and later the adult dog, to ride calmly and safely in a car. They keep the puppy from getting into mischief when no one is home to watch it, and for house-training they are essential. For show dogs they are a must.

Dogs usually won't mess in their special "houses," but left for long periods of time the puppy will break that rule, if necessary. Once that happens, the puppy will be much harder to train. To avoid accidents, and to use the crate properly, take the puppy out often, always after meals and after a nap, to a designated spot. Praise your puppy profusely for a job well done.

For messes in the house, a rebuke and a fast trip outside will give the pup the message. Harsh words, hitting with rolled-up news-

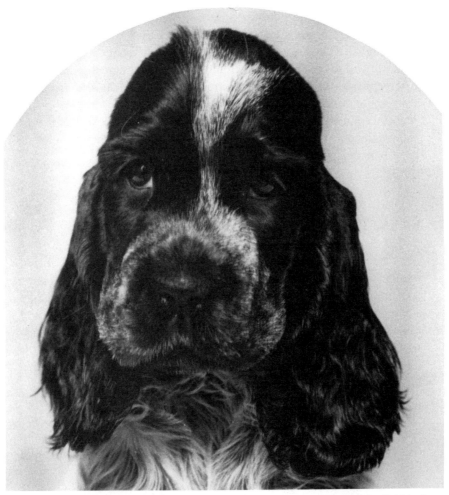

Ch. Aberdeen's Forget Me Not, blue roan puppy at three months (Ch. Kenobo Rabbit of Nadou ex Ch. Springfield's Maggie of Dunde).

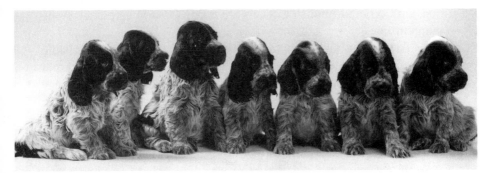

Puppies whelped in January 1988 by Ch. Daisymead's Dynasty ex Ch. Aberdeen's Forget Me Not.

papers, or wiping the puppy's nose in it will not solve the problem, but may create worse situations as time goes by.

English Cockers are generally very "soft" dogs. They do not respond well to yelling, loud scolding or physical abuse of any kind. After episodes of that type of correction, you will have a cringing, unhappy and unresponsive dog.

To train a dog takes time. To train an English Cocker takes time and gentleness. It is a breed that is anxious to please if they understand what is expected of them.

EARS, TEETH AND NAILS

Your puppy should be groomed regularly, and as part of that routine you should examine the inside of the ears. Long, floppy-eared dogs tend to develop infections if the ears are not kept clean. A little alcohol on a piece of cotton swabbed into the ear canal weekly should keep the ears dry and odor free. If you notice a dark, waxy substance when you clean the ears, you can suspect either a yeast infection or the presence of ear mites. Both are curable, but a trip to the veterinarian for proper diagnosis is important.

A puppy with ear problems may scratch its ears, shake its head often or try to rub the ears along the ground or against the furniture.

Treating ear problems as soon as they are noticed will save the dog from developing chronic ear infections, which are difficult, and sometimes impossible, to clear up.

As your puppy gets its second and permanent teeth, you can begin to introduce the toothbrush. Funny as it may seem, brushing a dog's teeth regularly, especially the rear molars, will keep breath sweet and prevent the development of plaque. Just as people get gum disease, dogs do, too, and English Cockers are prone to build up plaque along the gum line.

Toenail cutting is sometimes a chore that can develop into a battle between human and dog, but it need not be unpleasant if you start at a young age and do it regularly. Nails should be kept short (see page 39). When you hear them clicking on the floor they are too long. Some dogs' nails grow quickly and need to be done every couple of weeks, while others can go as long as a month before needing a trim. *Nails that are long will cause the puppy's feet to develop improperly, creating splayed feet and weak pasterns.*

EXTERNAL PARASITES

Weekly grooming also means checking for fleas, ticks and hot spots. English Cockers have a double coat, with the hair growing very thick next to the skin. This makes it difficult to spot parasites, but an itchy dog will give you a good idea that something is brewing under the coat. Prompt attention to any skin irritations (see page 39) will save massive problems later on. A dog that has skin problems, causing scratching and chewing, will never grow a good coat until the problems are resolved.

EXERCISE

The English Cocker is a Sporting dog, and therefore has the instinct to run and hunt. This does not mean that you should open the door and let your dog chase around the neighborhood. Responsible dog owners keep their pets under control at all times. A fenced yard will give your puppy room to play and stretch its legs. A game of catch with a rubber ball or a Frisbee is an excellent way for you and your dog to enjoy time together. A brisk walk on lead once or twice a day is another means you can use to get to know your pet, who will learn to look to you for good times.

Puppies should not be overtaxed, however. They should be allowed to exercise as much as they want, but not forced to do more than they are able. Puppies and adult dogs who get enough exercise will be calmer and quieter in the house and will not engage in destructive behavior.

SOCIALIZATION

From the time you bring your puppy home, it is beginning to learn social behavior. Observing and being part of the family will soon teach what is expected, and the dog will usually happily fit into the household.

A happy, outgoing, friendly dog will only result if you take the time to make the pup a family member. An English Cocker that is isolated away from people will never become a satisfactory pet. This breed quickly becomes shy, withdrawn and fearful unless exposed to different situations and people from an early age.

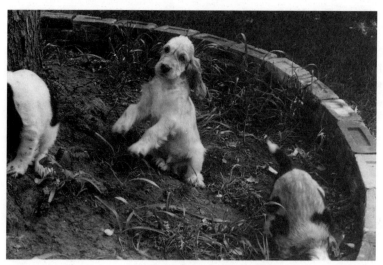

Eight-week-old puppies at play: orange roan Skylark's Pumpkin of Kenobo (Ch. Kvamme's Hollywood, TD, ex Skylark Free N Easy).

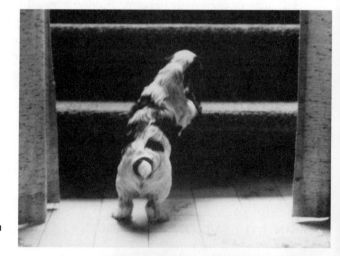

Stairs are a challenge for an eight-week-old puppy.

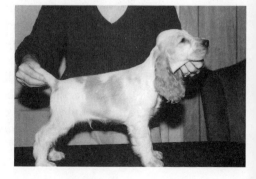

Three-month-old orange and white puppy, Encore's Am I Blue (Ch. Foxfyre Blue Blazer, CDX, ex Encore's Crystal Dawn).

30

Take your puppy walking, riding in the car, to the shopping center or park to meet other people and be exposed to other dogs in a controlled way. If you have a show puppy, take it to match shows; walk around the show grounds so the pup becomes familiar with the atmosphere.

Kindergarten puppy training, offered by some dog obedience clubs and schools, is an excellent way to socialize your pet without stress, while at the same time teaching you to train your dog.

ILLNESS

At the beginning of this chapter we said that three things are needed to develop a sound, healthy dog: time, attention and observation.

We have talked about the ways you need to spend time with your puppy and the attention that it needs. Observation is the third important ingredient.

You must know what is normal for your puppy: how much sleep, how much play, how many trips "to the bathroom," and what the pup looks like alert and awake. You need to observe normal behavior in order to determine when something is wrong.

The most obvious signs of a sick puppy are gastrointestinal. Diarrhea and vomiting are not symptoms that can be overlooked, but they are not the only signals that your dog is not up to par. Your puppy may be lethargic or sluggish, sleep more than usual or tire easily after a short time playing. Perhaps the pup has stopped eating. All these signs, some of which may be subtle, are indications that your pet is sick.

Illness becomes a medical emergency if the puppy becomes dehydrated, which can happen quickly in young dogs, if it runs a high fever or if you know that it has swallowed a poisonous substance. You must take it to the veterinarian *immediately* under any of these circumstances.

If the puppy does not seem to be recovering on its own after a couple of days of subnormal behavior, then it's off to the veterinarian for diagnosis and possible treatment. It is better to find out early, thereby eliminating the need for more expensive and lengthy treatment later on.

GENETIC DISORDERS OF THE ENGLISH COCKER

The English Cocker Spaniel is a natural breed. That is, it evolved from a functional hunting dog into the breed we see today without a great deal of genetic tinkering. It is a dog without the exaggerations that have led to problems in so many breeds. For example, the Pug and the Bulldog, with their pushed-in faces and awkward bodies, suffer from respiratory and reproductive problems. The German Shepherd Dog has a high incidence of hip dysplasia, partially incurred by its unstable hindquarters. Great Danes, because of their massive size, are prone to bone diseases, heart problems and a short life span.

The English Cocker has relatively few genetically programmed disorders. There are a few, however, and because of the relatively small gene pool with a limited number of dogs to breed from, they are difficult to eradiate.

Progressive Retinal Atrophy

Progressive retinal atrophy (PRA) is a degenerative disease of the retina in the eye. PRA is not unique to English Cockers. Several breeds are afflicted with one of the two forms of the disease, which are early onset and late onset. The early-onset form manifests itself as early as six months, and breeds prone to it, such as the Irish Setter and the Poodle, can be tested for the presence of the disease as early as four months.

English Cockers are not so lucky. They have the late-onset type of PRA, which does not begin to become evident until the dog is four or five years old. By that time, it has been shown, bred, and become an integral part of the family.

PRA is a recessive gene. It takes both parents carrying the gene to produce a blind puppy, though the parents themselves may not be blind. PRA can be carried along for several generations without ever expressing itself, until one carrier meets up with another carrier. Once that happens, both animals must be withdrawn from the breeding pool. Any offspring of those parents are suspect and should not be used for breeding, either. An affected dog should obviously never be bred.

PRA is a gradual process. The dog loses its night vision first and then eventually becomes completely blind. Blind dogs who are maintained in familiar surroundings do very well. As long as furniture is not moved around, and their usual habits are followed, they can live happy lives as companions.

Sometimes another dog in the household will watch over the handicapped. In one family the Irish Setter became the English Cocker's seeing eye dog, leading it outside, nudging it gently up or down the steps, and hovering over it to make certain it did not hurt itself.

There is no cure for PRA, although research has been ongoing for at least fifteen years to try to discover the cause. Now, with breakthroughs in genetic studies, it is possible that the gene causing PRA will be isolated and in time, perhaps, corrected. When that occurs, owners of the many breeds affected by this disease will be able to rejoice.

Epilepsy

Epilepsy is a neurological disease that affects many purebred and crossbred dogs. Idiopathic epilepsy—that is, epilepsy which has no known cause—is carried by many genes. It is polygenic, and is thought to be partially recessive. In research studies two epileptic dogs bred together will produce a much higher ratio of epileptic offspring than the normal population. However, there seems to be some evidence of one carrier being more dominant than another. At the current state of research into epilepsy it is practically impossible to predict who the carriers might be. However, a dog or bitch that has produced epileptic offspring should not be bred again, nor should any of the siblings in that litter. Epilepsy is not a serious problem in English Cockers, though it is occasionally seen.

There are many conditions that can cause seizures but are not classified as idiopathic epilepsy because a diagnosis can be found. Trauma, tumors, hormone imbalance, hypothyroidism, central nervous system disorders that affect the brain, all are possible reasons for a dog to have seizures. A thorough physical examination should be done as soon as the dog seizures the first time, to rule out all other possible causes before a diagnosis of true epilepsy can be made.

Epileptic dogs often develop a pattern of seizures. They may begin with one seizure a month, then progress over a period of time to twice a month, once a week and then more often. Sometimes dogs will have a cluster of seizures over two or three days and then be without them for an extended period.

After a dog has established an early pattern, it is possible to treat it with anticonvulsant drugs. English Cockers with idiopathic epilepsy can be maintained seizure free on a regimen of medication. Phenobarbitol is usually the drug of choice. The dog must be monitored frequently to be certain that the proper level of drugs is in the blood-stream, but with good veterinary care dogs can live normal lives for several years.

Renal Disease

Diseases of the kidneys are seen in several breeds, and in recent years there appears to be an increase of renal problems in the English Cocker. There seem to be two types of renal disease, both of which are genetically based.

Renal Cortical Hypoplasia. This is a disease characterized by in-sufficient development of the kidneys from the time the dog is quite young. Affected animals will show weight loss, stunted growth and increased thirst and urination. Eventually the dog will go into renal failure and die. Dogs with renal cortical hypoplasia can live several months or up to several years before the disease advances to the end stage.

Familial Nephropathy. Another similar disease is familial nephrop-athy, in which the kidneys are small and misshapen and do not develop as the dog grows. Dogs with this disease usually die before the age of two.

Both of these renal disorders are inherited, but the mode of in-heritance has not been established. It seems to run in a few bloodlines in the United States and in England. Dogs who have been known to produce renal disease in their offspring should be withdrawn from breeding.

Hip Dysplasia

Hip dysplasia is more commonly found in large, fast-growing breeds of dogs. However, it is sometimes seen in English Cockers, and for the most part breeders are conscientious about having their breeding stock radiographed before they are used.

Hip dysplasia is a polygenic malformation of the hip joint. Pup-pies are born with normal hips, but at some point, usually between the ages of six months and two years, changes in the fit of the ball of the hip into the socket occur. This causes abrasion to the bones, re-sulting in pain and lameness. Eventually arthritic changes are notice-able, and the dog will have difficulty getting up and down.

There are several procedures that can be surgically performed to relieve discomfort if the dog appears to be in chronic pain. Often a mild analgesic will suffice to keep the dog comfortable. English Cockers, however, do not suffer from hip dysplasia nearly to the degree that other breeds do, and if breeders continue to eliminate dysplastic dogs from their breeding programs, it will not become a widespread problem.

Other Abnormalities

Some other genetic abnormalities occur infrequently in English Cockers.

Hermaphroditism. Hermaphrodites—that is, puppies born with both male and female sex organs—are occasionally seen. The condition may be surgically corrected, but the dogs are probably infertile and should never be bred.

Vestigial Toes. Another problem has been surfacing during the past few years. Puppies are being born with one or two vestigial toes on one or more feet. The mode of inheritance is unknown, but if a bitch produces more than one of these puppies, she should not be used for breeding.

The responsibility of a breeder to protect the English Cocker cannot be overstated. Breeders are the backbone of the breed. Their concern for it and the ethics that they practice in producing sound, healthy puppies are essential for the future of the English Cocker as we know it.

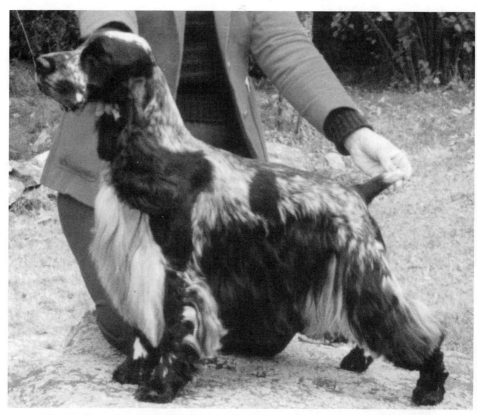

Ch. Cedarhurst Jonathan Seagull, beautifully groomed and ready for the show ring.

5

Grooming the English Cocker

The authors are indebted to Bonnie Threlfall, a breeder and professional handler who provided the demonstration and commentary for this chapter.

THE ENGLISH COCKER SPANIEL is a breed whose coat needs a great deal of attention in order to remain clean, unmatted and attractive. Left alone the coat will grow dense, sometimes curly, and will play host to a variety of brambles, burrs and external parasites. The English Cocker carries a double coat, long and silky on the outside, short and fine next to the skin. There are several types of coat found on the English Cocker, depending on the color and the lineage. Light particolors often carry a straight, silky coat which is easier to keep and groom than either the solid colors or the roans. Solids and roans tend to curl and grow longer, heavier coats, which mat easily and must be constantly brushed and combed.

Basic grooming involves keeping the dog clean, the nails clipped and the coat unmatted. Any good shampoo, including Ivory used for humans, is acceptable. Coat conditioner, such as Hagen oil, which is not rinsed out, helps to keep the coat free of tangles and split ends.

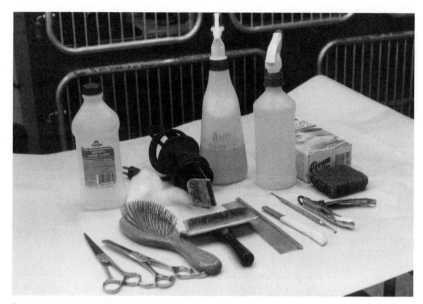

Grooming tools. *Rear, left to right:* Bottle of alcohol, cotton swabs, clippers, antistatic spray, coat conditioner spray, cornstarch, stripping stone. *Front, left to right:* Straight-edge shears, thinning shears, pin brush, slicker brush, comb, Real knife stripping blade, tooth scaler, nail clipper.

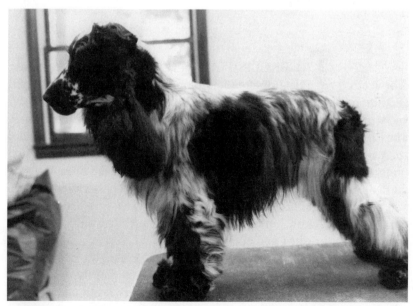

An English Cocker before it is groomed. This dog does not have a profuse coat, but it will take two to three hours to groom properly.

Any conditioner collects dirt after a few days, so the dog must be bathed weekly if conditioner is applied.

Fleas, ticks and other parasites can cause reactions that will destroy the coat and skin and make the dog miserable. Depending upon the climate and time of year, owners must be constantly vigilant and alert to any signs of unwelcome invaders. There are many dips, sprays and shampoos that can be used to rid the dog of these pests. Use only as directed and under the advice of your veterinarian.

Nails can be cut with a guillotine or scissors-type nail clipper, taking care that only the end and not the quick of the nail is cut. It is advisable to do the nails before anything else is done, in order to get that chore out of the way, so that once they are clipped the dog will relax for the rest of the session.

Most dogs enjoy being groomed once they are used to it. English Cockers should start being groomed early in life. Six weeks is about the time that they should begin to learn the routine that will be followed for most of their lives.

The first thing to teach them is to lie down on a grooming table. A grooming table can be anything from a kitchen table with a nonslip mat to a specially purchased table with a ridged rubber top. The table should be a height that is comfortable for the groomer. It should be sturdy enough so it does not wobble, causing the dog to be concerned about falling. Folding grooming tables can be purchased at pet supply outlets and are handy for storage and to carry to shows. They come in several sizes. In choosing one, make sure the dog can stretch out on it comfortably, as your English Cocker may need to be there for a couple of hours at a time.

GROOMING TOOLS

Grooming is made easier by using the proper tools. Listed are the tools needed to properly trim and prepare an English Cocker for the show ring.

Straight-edge Shears. Purchase good-quality, tempered-steel scissors and keep them sharp. These are used to edge around the feet, to do a last-minute touch-up on the whiskers and to trim the hair under the pads of the feet.

Single-edge Thinning Shears. These are used to blend the coat along the sides of the neck, around the feet and the base of the tail.

Clippers.   A good pair of clippers, such as the Oster professional small animal clipper in either the A2 or the A5 model, is essential for basic grooming. The blade most often used is the #10. It should be kept sharp, well lubricated and clean.

Pin Brush.   This is a brush with wire bristles set in a rubber base. It is used to separate the hair and to work out mats. This brush should not be used on the body of the dog as it might injure the skin. It is used on the feathers, working from the skin out to the ends of the hair in small sections. If mats are encountered, work them out with the fingers and the brush a few strands at a time.

Slicker Brush.   This is a wire brush with the ends of the wires bent. This brush can be used to go over the top coat and the ends of the ears. It should not be used on the feathers because it can break the hair.

Comb.   Use a metal comb with wide and narrow spacings. The comb is only used to go through the coat after it has been brushed, trimmed and bathed. Do not pull hair out with the comb or separate the feathers with the comb, as it will break the hair.

Stone.   The stripping stone is the tool you will use to do most of the trimming and shaping. It is a piece of porous rock that comes in the shape of a rectangle. It can be broken into smaller pieces to fit the hand and is used to pull out the undercoat and smooth the edges between the thinning shears and clippers.

Real Knife Stripper.   The stripping knife is used to remove dead hair and undercoat from the body. It is best used when it is slightly dull and is dragged through the coat with the grain of the hair.

Tooth Scaler.   English Cocker teeth tend to accumulate plaque, so along with the nail trim and general maintenance, scaling the teeth from the gumline down to the end of the tooth with a scaler will help preserve the teeth and prevent gum disease.

Alcohol and Cotton Swabs.   Keeping the ears clean is a vital part of good grooming as well as good health. Swabbing the ear canal gently with a cotton swab soaked in alcohol will help prevent wax buildup and yeast infections. This should be done weekly.

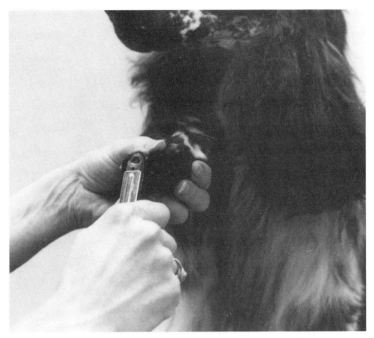

Cut the nails with a guillotine clipper.

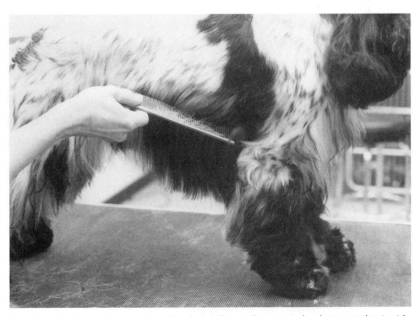

Imagine a line from elbow to tuck-up by placing the comb at an angle where you plan to strip.

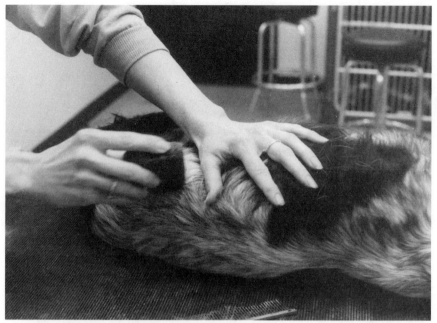

Strip the sides of the body using the same technique from thigh to shoulders.

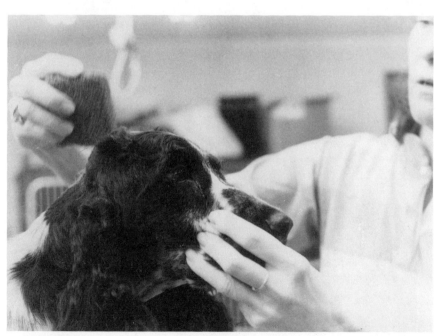

Strip the crown of the head as you did the body. Do not clip the top of the skull.

42

Antistatic Coat Spray. For finishing touches before going into the ring, spray the feathers with an antistatic spray to prevent flyaway ends.

Cornstarch. Cornstarch is sometimes used on the feathering to remove dirt and to give body to the coat. This is done at a show and is not a substitute for weekly bathing.

HOW TO TRIM YOUR ENGLISH COCKER FOR THE SHOW RING

There are several steps to trimming your English Cocker for show. They involve stripping, clipping and scissoring, which must be done in sequence to achieve the desired effect.

When stripping dead and unwanted hair from the dog, it is best to do it when the dog has not been freshly bathed. A good time frame would be to strip the coat four days prior to a show. Bathe the dog and do the clipping three days before the show; touch up and rebathe just before the show. After the dog has been bathed for the final time, blanket the coat and leave it blanketed until just before entering the ring.

Stripping

It usually takes two to three hours to strip a dog that has not been trimmed regularly. Lay the dog down on the table on its stomach and work from the tail toward the head up the middle of the back. Lift the hair with your hand in the opposite direction from the way it grows. With the stone in your other hand, pull the hair down. You do not go over the hair you have just done. You will be pulling out the hair in layers without pulling the topcoat. Work your way from just in front of the base of the tail to the base of the skull.

Next lay the dog on one side and do the same thing from the thigh to the shoulders. Turn the dog over and do the other side. Ideally, when you are finished with the stripping you should see no hair sticking out. The feathering and all the body coat should be "molded" to the dog.

When doing the sides, start below the widest part of the body so the feathering will lie close to the dog and not stick out. Go with the lines of the dog at an angle from the elbow to the tuck-up. The line

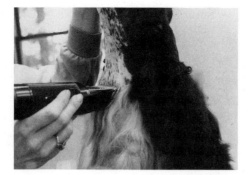

Clip the hair against the grain from a spot just below the widest part of the neck up to the chin.

Clip the sides of the face against the grain. Do not clip above the level of the eye.

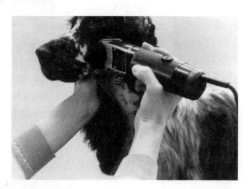

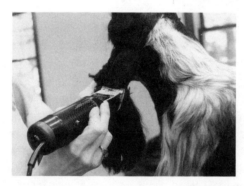

Clip up the ears against the grain.

Clip the hair on the ear burr.

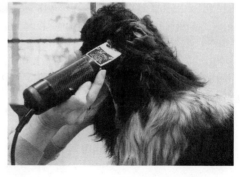

from elbow to tuck-up continues to the front between the legs. Use the spine of your comb as a guideline, laying the comb along the body and stripping above that line. The hair should be shaped so the dog does not look low and dumpy. Each dog is individual, and you must have a picture in your mind of how you want the dog to appear once it is done.

To strip the top of the skull, stand the dog up and use the stone just as you did along the body. Leave enough hair on the top of the head so the planes of the head appear to be parallel.

Clipping the English Cocker for the Show Ring

After you have stripped the coat and shaped the body hair the way you think it looks best, you will be ready to use the clipper. A clipper is not a substitute for stripping and should only be used in certain areas: the sides of the head, the neck, the ears and under the feet.

Working up just below the widest part of the neck, clip the hair against the grain all the way to the chin, using a #10 blade. Stretch the lip back to clip out the hair in the folds of the lower lip. Clip up the sides of the throat to the lower jaw. The individual planes of the dog's head will determine where you should clip the face. If you clip "the stop" too far down the nose, the dog will appear down-faced and scowling. If you begin the stop too far up, they will look surprised. Before taking the blade to the face, mark the stop with a V which you make with your scissors. Then clip against the grain. Once the hair is removed from the stop and cheeks, clip *with* the grain just to blend to the point of the V.

When you are clipping the sides of the face, do not go above the eye line. Clip as close as possible on the muzzle to show off the chiseling, but do not clip up to the head. Use the clipper on its edge under the eye and along the muzzle. Leave some hair around the foreface to give a "plushy" soft look. In order to make the planes as parallel as possible, leave hair to create the illusion of a rectangle.

The feathering on the ears should just clear the underline of the jaw, so you are not adding any bulk to the jaw when you look at the dog head on. Mark your spot on the ears where you will begin to clip by making a V with your scissors. Clip up the ears above the V against the grain. Take the hair on the inside of the ears as far down as the outside to allow air to get into the ears for health reasons. Clip off the hair on the ear burr. Lift the ear and go down the ridge of hair on

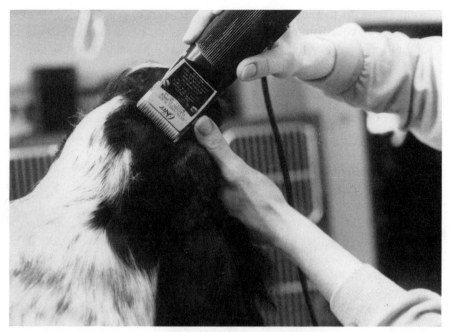

Clip a circle behind the ear, taking care not to clip into the hair on the back of the neck.

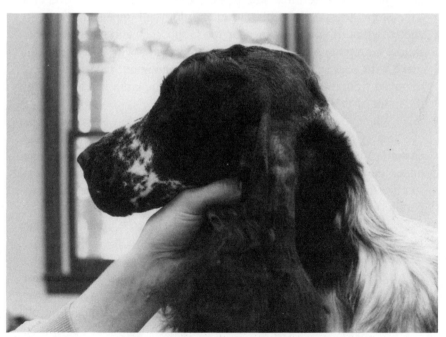

Muzzle and ear after clipping.

46

the neck holding the edge of the clipper farthest away from you against the hair. Run the clipper down the ridge of hair and stop where you stopped clipping the throat.

Clip *with* the grain along the sides of the head right above the ear. Do not clip the occiput or the back skull. Clip only to the eye-ear line. Clip a circle behind the ear with the back edge of the clipper against the base of the ear, taking care not to clip into the hair on the back.

Next, scoop out the hair under the feet with the clippers in order to remove mats. Shape around the big pad, but do not clip the top of the foot. The rest of the trimming is done with the thinning shears.

Scissoring

Once you have gone over the dog with the stone and the clippers, you will be ready to use the single-blade thinning shears.

The shears are used to blend the hair where the clipper has left delineating lines. First, thin the hair on the top of the head and the back skull so the head appears rectangular and with no sharp edges where the clippers have been used. Next, use the shears with the grain of the hair along the sides of the neck, taking the hair down as close as possible. Accentuate the shoulder angulation by trimming the sides, but without cutting into the chest hair. Outline the shoulder and the leg by first separating the leg hair from the chest and then scissoring. Blend the hair by using a comb along the sides, lifting the coat up and cutting on top of the comb. When you are finished you should not see any seams; one area should blend into the other so the dog looks as if it was born that way. Once you have done the shoulders with the shears, you should be able to keep it up with the stone, providing it is done weekly.

Do not thin the shoulder hair with the scissors. All thinning and stripping is done with the stone, pulling out hair from underneath.

The foot of the English Cocker should be small, round and high-toed, looking as much like a cat's paw as possible. To shape the foot, be sure there are no mats between the toes. Keep the bottom edge of the thinning shears on the table, and go around the foot as close to the foot as possible. Try to avoid picking up the other foot, as it will cause the foot bearing the weight to splay. Put a little pressure on the other elbow to get the dog to stand on the foot being trimmed. Keep going around the foot with the blade on the table until you get nothing off. Pick up the foot and take out the hair underneath, taking care not

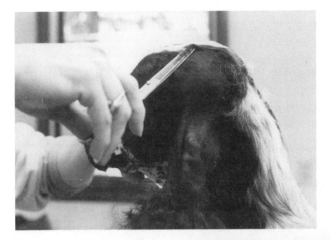

Thin the hair on top of the head and back skull with thinning shears.

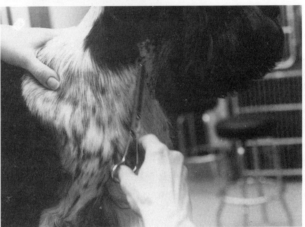

Use the shears with the grain along the sides of the neck.

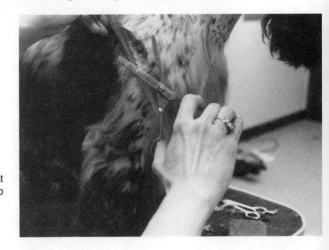

Blend the hair by lifting the coat with the comb and cutting on top of the comb.

48

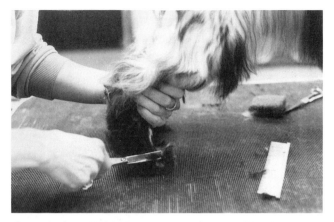

Shape the foot with thinning shears with the edge of the blade resting on the table.

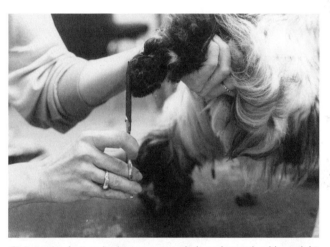

Pick up the foot and take out excess hair underneath with straight-edge shears.

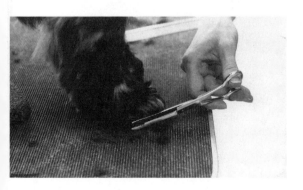

Finish off the foot with straight-edge shears as you did with the thinning shears.

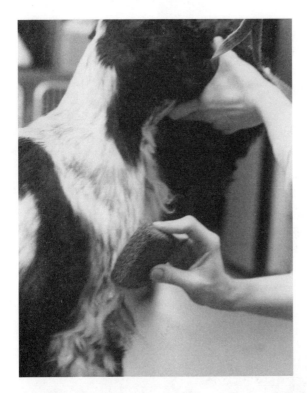

Once you have done the shoulders with
the shears, you can maintain the coat
by stripping weekly with the stone.

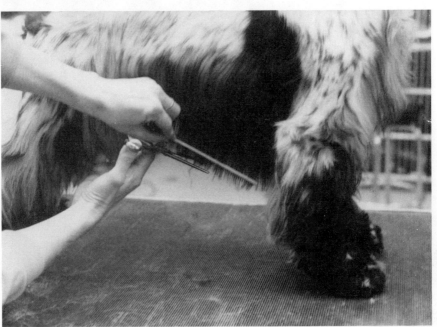

The line of the feathering should follow the tuck-up.

50

to cut the pads or take too much hair out between the toes. You do not want to see individual toes when the dog is standing. Once you have taken off as much as possible with the thinning shears, go around the foot again with a straight-edge scissors, using the same technique with the blade resting on the table.

Looking at the dog from the front, you should not see any hair sticking out along the sides. Hair on the inside of the front legs should be trimmed even with the chest bone. Trim off the hair on the sides of the front legs so that no hair is flying out of the sides when the dog moves. Shape the chest feathering so the lowest point of the feathering is right between his legs, and so that it comes to a point. The feathering should follow the dog's natural conformation, with the line of the feathering following the tuck-up. The dog should not appear dumpy. That means if the dog has a profuse coat in front, it should be trimmed in proportion to the belly coat. When trimming the feathers you should take into account the show conditions. For indoor shows you would let the hair grow longer. For outdoor shows you would trim it higher so the dog does not look dumpy in the grass.

Trim in a straight line from the tuck-up to the top of the leg. You can make the dog look shorter or longer in back by trimming the tuck-up further forward or rearward.

Trim the back feet just as you did the front, but do not lift the hair away from the top of the foot or the dog will look as if it is wearing shorts. Trim the hocks on an angle with the back pad. The hair will be cut closer near the foot. Pull the hair around to the side of the hock and take off the hair on both the inside and the outside of the hock, trimming closer on the inside.

Trim around the tail, taking off all the excess hair, but avoid cutting into the body. Blend the hair under the tail and scissor about halfway down the leg to the widest part of the second thigh. You do not want to see any hair sticking out of the sides of the upper legs or thighs. When you trim the feathering on the front of the thigh, shape it to just uncover the top of the foot and blend with the feathering on the belly.

Once you have trimmed with the thinning shears, go over the dog with the stone, blending in all the rough edges and pulling out flyaway hairs. Use the stone to blend the scissoring and the clipping on the head and neck so that no lines appear. Then take the Real stripper and drag the coat with the grain to remove any additional dead hair from the back and sides.

After you have finished, bathe the dog for the final time before

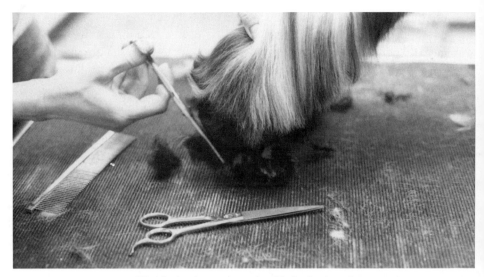

Trim the hocks on an angle with the back pad.

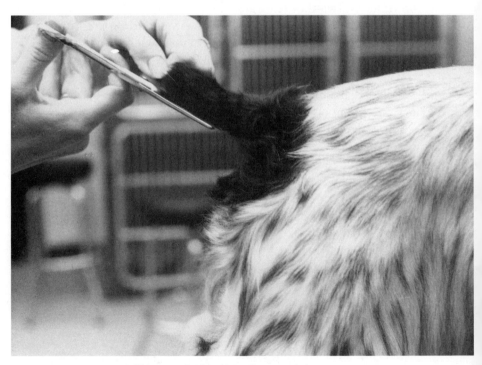

Trim around tail, taking off excess hair.

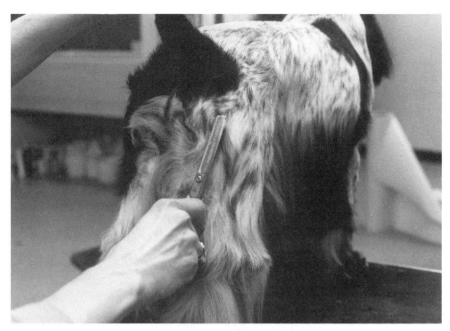

Blend hair under the tail and scissor halfway down the leg.

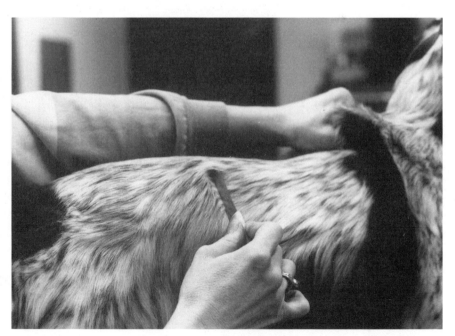

Take Real stripper and, with the blade lying flat against the coat, drag the coat with the grain to remove additional dead hair.

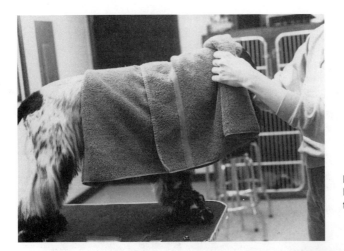

Fold a terry-cloth bath towel in half and double-fold it around the neck, forming a collar.

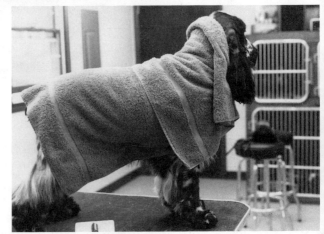

Blanketed dog ready to go to the show.

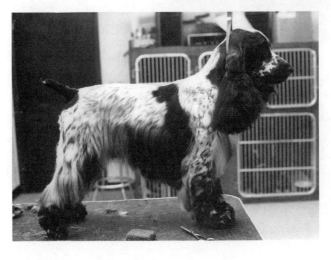

Finished dog ready to be shown.

the show and wrap him in a blanket. While the dog is wet, brush the coat down with a pin brush. Take a terry cloth bath towel large enough to be folded over but not so big that it drags on the ground when you are done. Fold the towel in half and then double-fold it around the neck of the dog, making a collar that will not slide down the neck. Hold the dog's head out, not up, and pin the blanket horizontal to the dog with a horse-blanket pin. Pin it snugly enough that it cannot move. Make sure the body coat is lying flat and pin the blanket under the loin horizontally.

Now your dog is ready for the show.

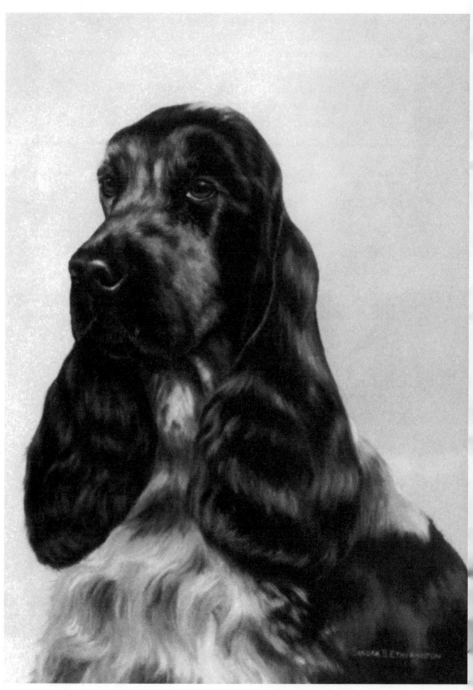

An oil portrait by Sandra B. Etherington of Ch. Olde Spice Sailor's Beware. "Dusty" is the top winning bitch in breed history. Her accomplishments include an unprecedented three National Specialty Best of Breed wins.

56

6

Showing the
English Cocker

ENGLISH COCKERS are, above all, lovable pets, but you may decide to attend a local dog show just to see if you would like to participate with your dog in this hobby. Perhaps the breeder from whom you purchased your dog has encouraged you to show it, because their experience has told them that your purchase has "show potential."

Sometimes breeders will sell a promising puppy to a pet home on the condition that it be shown, at least a few times, to see if it lives up to its early promise.

There are two basic kinds of dog shows that are held throughout the United States. One is the "match show." This is an informal way of introducing puppies and inexperienced handlers to the intricacies of dog showing. There are no championship points awarded at matches, but they are usually conducted according to AKC regulations.

The other is the "point show," at which AKC championship points are awarded according to the number of dogs competing in any particular breed on that day. The point schedule is made up by the AKC each year and varies within nine regions throughout the United States. "Specialty shows" are point shows also, but are for one breed only. The English Cocker Spaniel Club of America holds a National Specialty show each year that rotates to different parts of the country.

Local English Cocker Spaniel clubs hold shows and matches throughout the year. The American Kennel Club can give you the name of the local club nearest you.

Dog showing can be a very enjoyable pastime for the whole family, but it does take some preparation and experience in order to get the most benefits from it. The experience will come with practice and by watching handlers in the rings with their dogs.

Showing has a certain ritual to it. The procedures are relatively simple. You enter certain classes according to the dog's age, sex and maturity. Point shows are entered in advance; most matches are entered the day of the event. A set routine is followed in the ring. As you enter in a line, you will pose your dog, called "stacking" or "setting up your dog," for the judge's initial inspection. When the judge has marked everyone present and has looked over the class, he or she will ask the class to gait around the ring once or twice. Then the judge will examine each dog individually. English Cockers are examined on a table, so the judges do not have to kneel on the ground to see each one. After the judge looks at your dog from head to tail you will be asked to gait the dog. You will either go straight down to the end of the ring and back to the judge, or you will make a triangle, according to the judge's instructions. After all the dogs in the class have been examined, the judge usually asks the class to go around together once more. Then the judge will make selections, placing them one through four.

After all the classes for non-champions have been judged, males separately from females, the judge will pick a Winners Dog and a Winners Bitch from among the first place winners in each class. Winners Dog and Winners Bitch win the points, from one point (being the least) up to five points, which are awarded at shows with large entries.

Following the selection of Winners Dog, Winners Bitch and a Reserve winner to each of these, the Specials are called into the ring. These are dogs who have already won their championships. They will compete, along with Winners Dog and Winners Bitch, for Best of Breed and Best of Opposite Sex to Best of Breed. The Winners Dog and Winners Bitch are also reexamined for Best of Winners.

All of this may seem confusing, but once you have observed at several shows, the routine will fall into place. Before you ever set foot in a ring yourself, it is imperative that you watch how the dogs are set up, gaited and handled in the ring. After a few shows you should begin to develop what experienced dog fanciers call "an eye for a dog." That is, you will be able to discern what makes some dogs

58

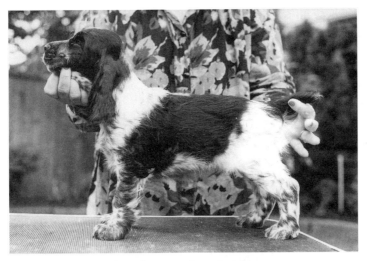

Learning to stack on the table.

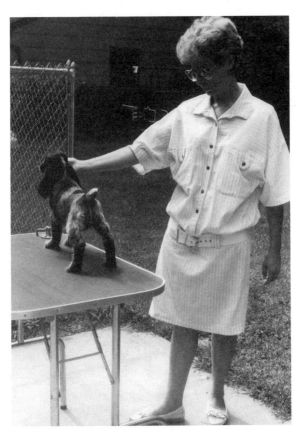

From the rear.

better show dogs than others. Not everyone, of course, has the powers of observation or the knowledge to be a true dog fancier, but you will never know unless you try.

THE MAKING OF A SHOW DOG

What makes a great show dog? First of all, it must have most of the characteristics that are described in the Standard. It should not have major flaws in structure. Then, it must have a "look-at-me" attitude, which becomes evident as it walks with its head held high, tail wagging with an alert, friendly expression.

Structure is nurtured by proper care, nutrition and exercise. The attitude must be developed with equal diligence from the time the puppy is small. English Cockers are notorious for preferring to chase birds or lie on the couch, rather than trot around a show ring. You must make showing fun at the same time you are teaching them to gait on a show lead and stand quietly on the ground or on a table.

There are a few pieces of equipment that you must have to become a true show-goer. The first is a grooming table. These are collapsible, rubber-topped tables at the proper height for either grooming your English Cocker or practicing the stack. This is the same kind of table that judges use in the ring, so you must get your puppy accustomed to standing up high off the ground. Grooming tables also are essential to save your own back as you do the regular coat, nails and ears maintenance.

Grooming tables and all other dog show and dog care accessories are available at concessionaires at most dog shows, or through mail-order catalogs or pet supply houses.

You will need a show lead. This is a thin lead made of nylon, leather or treated fabric that slips over the dog's head. You will have to practice putting the lead on and taking it off quickly, without getting yourself and the dog entangled. Some people prefer a thin choke chain rather than a slip collar, but this will depend on how your dog reacts to each. Some dogs move better on a loose lead. Others need the control of a choke. You should experiment with both.

When you set up your dog on the table or on the floor, it is useful to practice in front of a mirror, so you can see how the dog looks from the judge's point of view. It is also helpful to ask someone with experience to show you the basic steps. You will find most dog fanciers willing to help the novice get started.

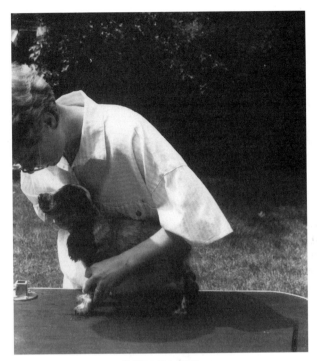

Setting the front.

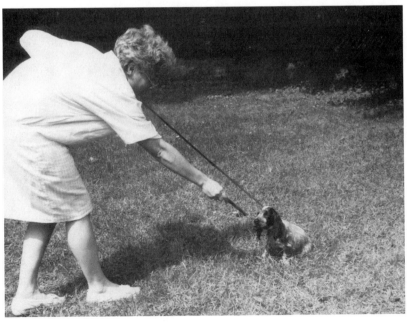

A little encouragement.

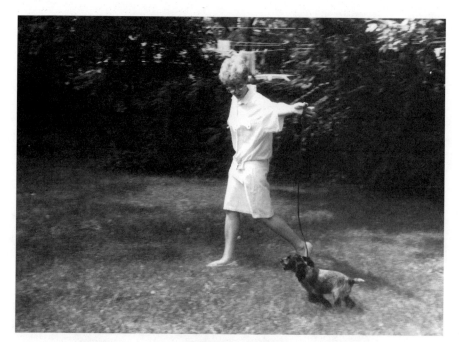

Full speed ahead.

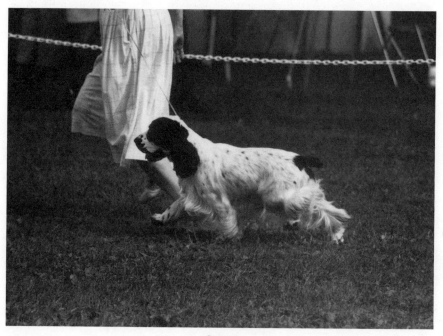

Gaiting.

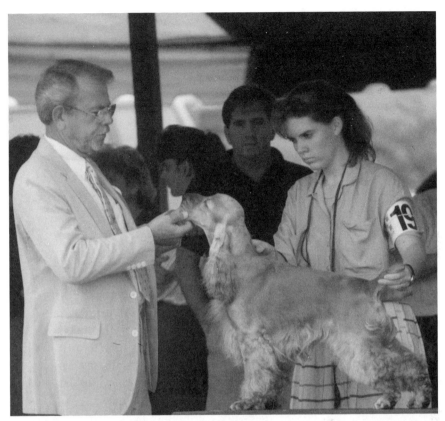

The real thing—stacking for the judge and standing for examination. Junior handler Jennifer Alston shows her dog Ricky.

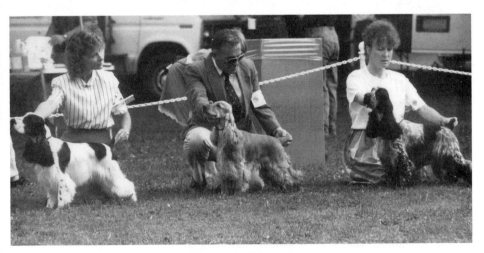

Stacking on the ground.

63

Some dog clubs offer show handling classes, and these are very useful to accustom you and your dog to the show ring before you venture out for the real thing.

You will need all the customary paraphernalia for grooming your English Cocker and a small kit or box, such as a tack box, to carry to shows. Brush, comb, spray bottle with water or conditioner, talc or cornstarch to give body to the feathers, scissors and stone for last-minute trimming. You will also need to take fresh water and a bowl, possibly the most important items for the comfort of your English Cocker.

One essential piece of equipment is a crate. The same one you used to house-train your puppy is fine to put into the car to take to shows. With the dog in a crate you can leave all the windows open without fear that it will escape. If it is a hot or rainy day and you would like to be close to the ring, you can place your crate under the show tent near your ring. Your dog will have a comfortable place to stay while you watch other classes. Keeping your English Cocker in a crate at the show enables it to rest and not become worn out trekking around the grounds until it is time to perform. Too often one sees an owner walking a puppy around for hours until it is time to go into the ring. By then the puppy is exhausted, the owner is frustrated because it won't look alive, the judge ignores it and an entry fee has been wasted.

Crates, tack boxes, water jugs, grooming tables, chairs or even one's own exercise pen have made show-goers the ultimate "schleppers." Call it common sense, or the tricks of the trade; most of what they carry serves to make a day at the show more comfortable for dogs and owners.

PROFESSIONAL HANDLERS

Dog shows are the only organized sport in which amateurs and professionals compete against one another. This does not mean that the professionals always win. This is especially true in English Cockers, a breed that is primarily shown by their owners. In fact, the National Specialty has been won three times by the same owner with the same bitch, Vicky Spice with her Ch. Olde Spice Sailors Beware.

There are good reasons for hiring a professional handler. Some people, after trying it themselves, find it just too wearing, or they may find that they really are so clumsy that they are tripping over themselves and their dog. Dog showing also is a time-consuming hobby, and unless one is willing to devote many weekends, indoors and out, in all kinds of weather, a professional handler may be needed.

Professionals charge fees, which may vary from handler to handler. As in every business, a few are very good, most are average, and a few are terrible. If you decide to give your English Cocker to a professional, you will have to do your homework to find the right person for you, one who knows English Cockers and how to groom, care for and show them to their best advantage. Talk to other English Cocker fanciers, especially those who use handlers, to get opinions about them. Use your own powers of observation to determine who seems to be knowledgeable about the breed. Take the time to find just the right person for your dog and then give it a trial run.

English Cocker fanciers are for the most part a relaxed and friendly group of people. The vast majority show their dogs themselves because it is a pleasant hobby, a way to get together with their dogs and other English Cocker lovers. Everyone goes with the hope that their dog is the one to win on that day, but if they lose they are usually good sports and if they win they are, for the most part, gracious and courteous.

JUNIOR SHOWMANSHIP

Classes are held for children at many shows. In these classes the youngsters are judged on how well they show their dogs and on their ring manners. English Cockers are good for juniors to show because they are small enough to be manageable and are patient enough to put up with fumbling fingers. Several good handlers and breeders of English Cockers began their careers in junior showmanship.

Children are eligible to compete from the age of ten to the age of eighteen. They are divided into classes by age and by experience into junior and senior categories. They will compete in classes with all breeds of dogs, except at Specialty shows, where only English Cockers are entered.

Children who are interested in showing dogs gain valuable lessons in sportsmanship and responsibility. If they must care for their English Cocker themselves, they will learn how to treat the animal properly and the dog will form a special bond with its young handler. Parents can encourage youngsters to participate in shows as part of a family endeavor, thereby making dog showing truly a family affair.

Showing a dog brings out the best and sometimes the worst in

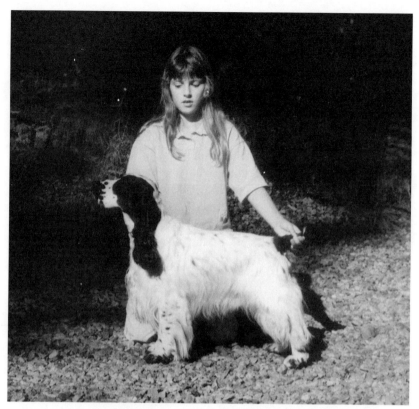

A junior practicing at home: Jessica Dufford and "Chip."

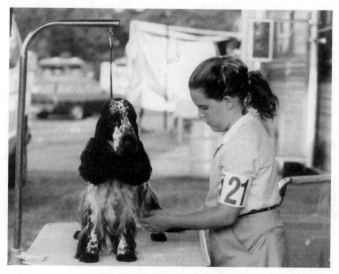

Juniors must learn to groom.

people. Those who go to enjoy themselves and their dogs in the company of friends will get much more out of this hobby than those who go only to win. In any competition there are good days and bad, and one must be willing to be a good loser as well as a gracious winner. Good sportsmanship reflects well on you and your dog, especially since judging a dog is such a subjective thing. One judge may perceive a dog as the best representative of the Standard one day, and the next day that same dog may lose because another judge is of a different opinion.

Win or lose, the English Cocker you took to the show is the same one you are taking home. If the dog was good enough in your eyes to bring, it should be no different whether or not you carry home a blue ribbon.

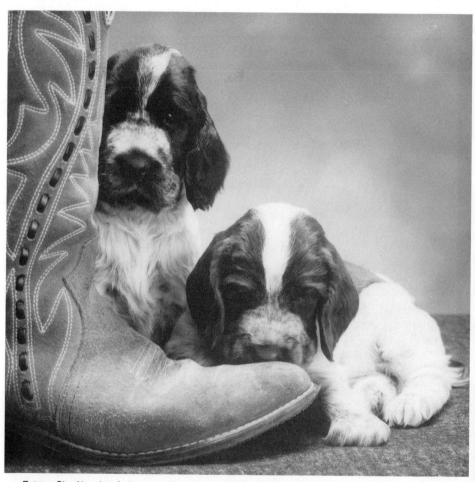

Future Ch. Aberdeen's Lyssa of Wyndsor and Aberdeen's Tam O'Shanter getting a toehold on their world.

7

Breeding the English Cocker

THERE COMES A TIME in almost every owner's life when the idea of breeding that wonderful English Cocker bitch comes to mind.

It may be that you bought your puppy "on breeder's terms." That means that the breeder will decide when and to whom your precious English Cocker will be bred. If that is the case, then your decision will have already been made. You will also have the benefit of the breeder's experience when it comes time to whelp the litter.

It may also be that you bought a puppy as a pet, on limited registration. In that case, it cannot be bred because the puppies will be unregistrable, and therefore you need think no more about it. Responsible breeders use only breeding stock that is able to be registered with the American Kennel Club.

If neither of the above conditions prevail, as an owner you have some serious thinking to do. The first question to be answered is whether your bitch is really of good enough quality to breed. You may think she is the most gorgeous creature on earth, but does she come close to the Standard for English Cockers? You should seek the advice of a couple of knowledgeable breeders before you proceed further.

If it is determined that "yes" she is of breeding quality, the next question is "why?" **Here are some reasons NOT to breed your bitch:**

It would be good for her to have one litter before she is spayed. This is a medically incorrect position. It makes no difference to her if she bears a litter or not. And, if you decide that she will only have one litter, she runs less of a risk of getting mammary cancer if she is spayed at a young age.

We want the children to witness the birth of puppies. Children usually have only a fleeting interest and are gone to other activities, leaving you with the care and the bills that a litter brings.

We know so many people who want one of her pups. Don't believe it. Those interested parties always vanish the minute you announce the birth of your litter.

We want one just like her. That's closer to a reason, but don't depend upon it. Dogs no not generally replicate themselves, because they are genetically too diverse. To approximate this desire, you would have to breed very closely and carefully within her line.

Her puppies will pay for the cost of buying her. That is never a good excuse. To do it right will cost you far more than the price of the bitch to begin with. Just for starters, the stud fees start at $350.00. Then there is the prenatal exam, shots for the puppies, dewclaw and tail docking expenses, plus the expenses for advertising the puppies for sale. These routine costs do not include complications, such as Caesarean sections or sick puppies.

To make money on one litter is a rare occurrence. One has to have a long history of breeding good puppies, so that buyers are waiting for your next litter, before you will see any profit in this hobby.

What, then, are the reasons to breed an English Cocker litter? If you are seriously interested in the breed, and strive to improve what you have, then producing a litter is an exciting adventure.

If you want to keep a puppy, either of the same sex or the opposite, then breeding it yourself creates a special bond to that newcomer. This is not the same thing as trying to find a duplicate of what you have.

If you have become interested in the world of purebred dogs, then breeding your first litter is a good way to continue in the sport.

GOING AHEAD

Once the decision has been made, well ahead of your bitch's next season you must seek the advice of a reputable breeder. If you have

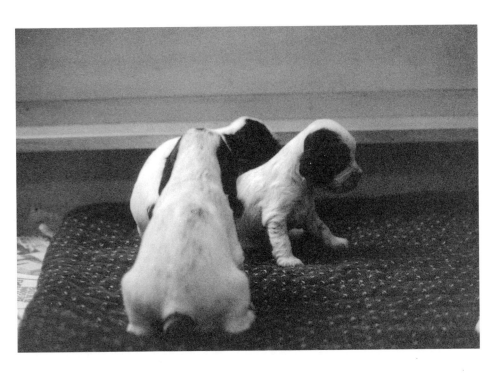

English Cocker puppies at three and a half weeks.

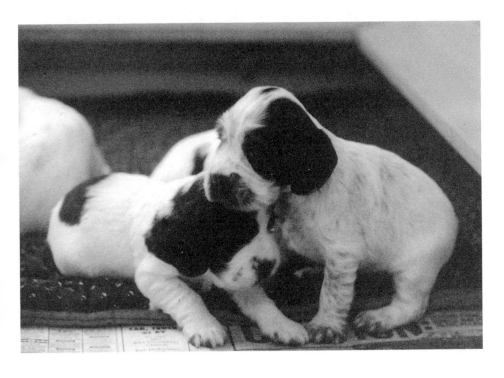

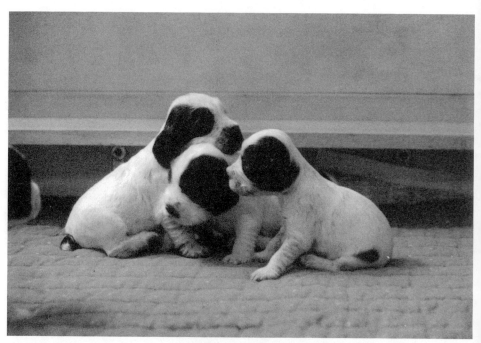

The committee meets . . .

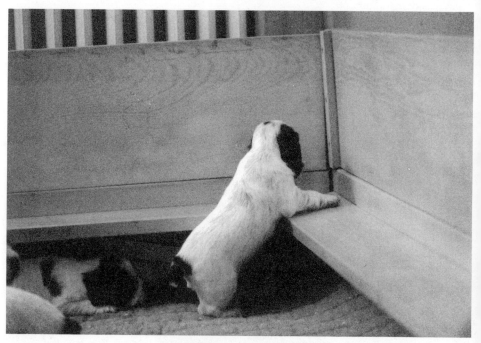

. . . and decides to send out a scout!

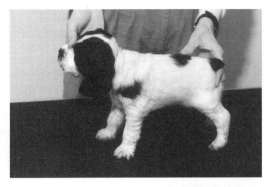

English Cocker puppy at four weeks.

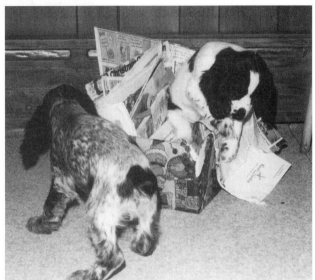

English Cocker puppies at eight weeks—the paper chase!

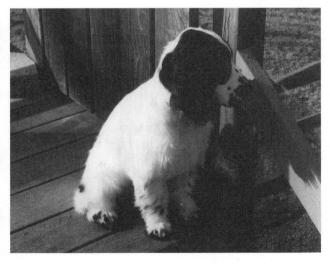

English Cocker puppy at four months.

maintained contact with the person from whom you bought the bitch, that is a good place to start. He or she can advise you on a suitable mate, and if willing, can guide you through the whole process. If that contact is not an option, seek out and join a local English Cocker club to meet the breeders, and attend some local shows, where you can watch the dogs being judged. You may find a stud just right for your bitch.

Before going further, your bitch should be radiographed to be sure she is free of hip dysplasia, and her eyes must be checked by a veterinary ophthalmologist to be certain she does not have PRA. She must be free of internal and external parasites and be in optimum health. Before she is bred all her vaccinations should be current; you should not vaccinate or give any medications while she is in whelp. Only then should you approach the owner of a prospective sire.

When you have chosen a mate, you should have a written contract with the owner. You should know in advance what the stud fee will be, how many services will be provided for that fee and whether the owner of the stud wants to be paid at the time of service or when the puppies are born. Occasionally, the owner of the sire will take a puppy instead of a stud fee. Other possibilities are that the stud fee be paid half at the time of the breeding and the rest when the litter is born. Some stud owners only ask a fee if more than two live puppies result from the mating. There are many variations, but the terms should be clearly understood by both parties and contracted for on paper.

COLOR GENETICS

English Cockers come in so many different colors that you may want to try to select a sire that will give you a variety. Here's where a basic knowledge of genetics comes in. To give yourself better odds you would have to know the color patterns of most of the antecedents in the pedigrees of both your bitch and her chosen mate. Even then, there are often surprises in an English Cocker whelping box.

Solid-color dogs, either red or black, are the easiest to determine. Solid coloring is always dominant to roans or open marked partis; black is dominant to all other colors. If one of the parents is black, each puppy in that litter has at least a 50 percent chance of being black.

Red is recessive to black. This means that it takes two reds bred together to produce all reds. However, reds may result from a mating

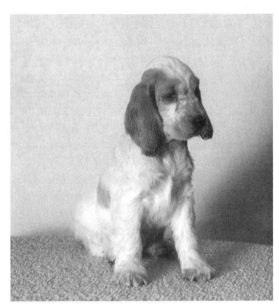

From puppy to adult: Ch. Kvammes High Style, orange roan (Ch. Olde Spice Crusader ex Ch. Kvammes Razzle Dazzle). *Top:* At eight weeks; *Bottom:* as an adult.

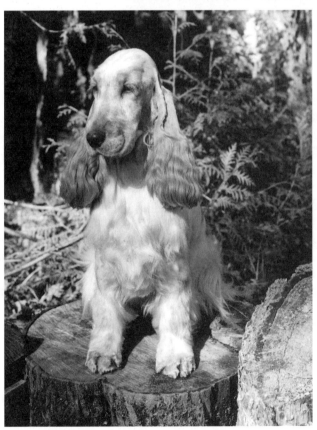

of two blacks if both black parents carry the recessive red gene. If a red is bred to a black that carries a recessive red gene, half of the litter may be red. If the black parent does not carry the red gene, all of the puppies will be black.

Black and tan and liver and tan are solid colors that are recessive. It takes both the sire and the dam carrying the tan factor to produce either combination. Liver is the one color other than black that can produce black when bred to a color other than black. Liver bred to liver will produce only liver.

Solids are dominant to roans and roans are dominant to white ticked and to open marked particolors. The colors are inherited in partis and roans according to the same rules as solids. A black that carries two particolor genes will be black and white. If it carries a roan gene it will be blue roan. A red with two particolor genes will be orange and white or orange roan.

Blue roaning comes in many shades, with the darker colors generally dominant to the lighter roans. An orange roan dog bred to a black and white, for instance, may produce some dark roans, because the black and white is dominant to the orange or red gene.

Breeding solids to roans or particolors is generally not done, because mismarks may result. This would be a solid dog with white paws, or large asymmetrical patches that are not pleasing to the eye. In breedings such as this, some of the litter will be solid and *all* will henceforth carry the parti factor. Solids resulting from breeding solid to parti are called hybrid solids.

Tri markings—that is, black, white and tan, or blue roan and tan—are the result of a recessive gene that can attach itself to any color but needs to find the same recessive in its mate to express itself.

When looking at newborn puppies, if the nose and footpads are black the puppy will be a blue roan. If they are pink, or pink with black flecks, the result will be black and white, or black and white ticked. Ticking and light roaning do not emerge until the puppies are several weeks old, so you may think you have a clear black and white, or orange and white, litter, but will be surprised at the changes as the puppies grow.

ANTICIPATING THE LITTER

Once your bitch has been bred, she needs to maintain a good regimen of exercise and care. She can remain on her regular diet until

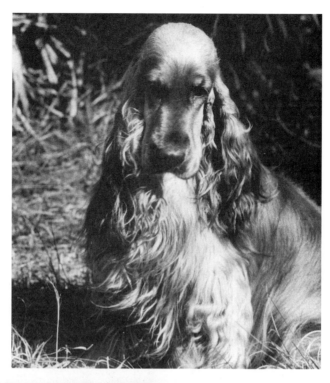

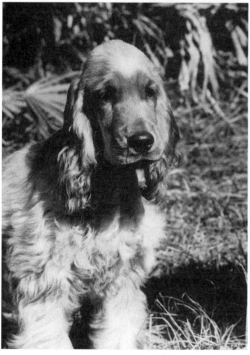

Father and son: Ch. Rustlin Dauntless Diplomat *(top)* and Rustlin Surprise Sunset *(bottom)*, reds.

77

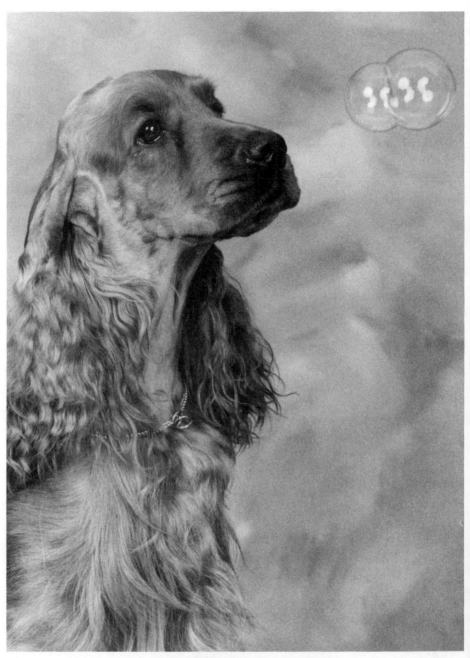

Rustlin Surprise Sunset as an adult.

about halfway through her pregnancy, when her food intake should be increased by about one third.

As her term nears (between fifty-eight and sixty-three days from the time of her first breeding), be aware of any unusual vaginal discharges or obvious discomfort. You should be able to feel the puppies moving inside her abdomen, unless there are only one or two, in which case they are difficult to detect. Her nipples should begin to swell and become pink, and if she is carrying a number of puppies she may become ungainly. Anything from five to eight puppies is considered a normal litter for English Cockers.

English Cockers are usually easy whelpers once the first puppy has arrived, but you still should already have established a good working relationship with your veterinarian. The possibility for trouble always exists, and you may need medical assistance in a hurry.

As the bitch's term approaches, you should prepare a whelping box for her. This can be anything from a sturdy cardboard box to a wooden box to a plastic wading pool lined with papers and soft cloths. Introduce her to the box several days ahead so she will become accustomed to her new quarters. English Cockers love to have their puppies on your bed, under the bed or in your closet, so you will have to keep your eye on her at the first signs of restlessness, panting or digging in dark corners.

A complete treatise on breeding and whelping a litter is beyond the purview of this book, but there are some good self-help books about the subject in print. One of the best is *The Joy of Breeding Your Own Show Dog* by Anne Serrane (New York: Howell Book House, 1980). If you have to do it alone, this one book will help you through it step by step.

In all aspects of raising an English Cocker, from puppyhood through motherhood, care and management are primarily a matter of common sense. One must appreciate the breed for what it is. Working with people you trust, you can raise puppies that will become sound and healthy adults.

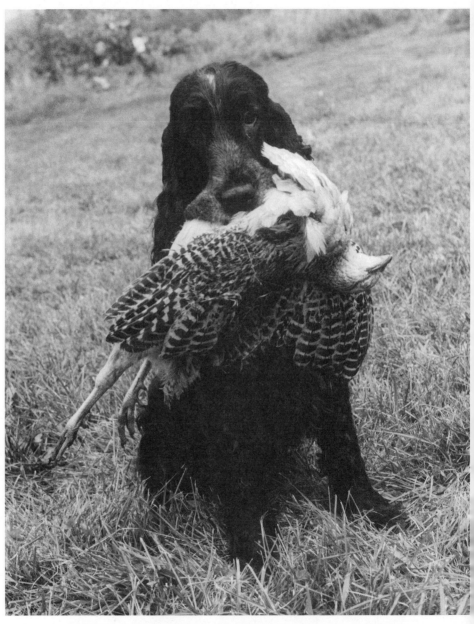

Log Tavern Lad of Meadowrue, CD, WDX, shows how he earned his titles.

8

English Cockers in the Field

T HE FIRST field trial for Cocker Spaniels was held in the autumn of 1925 under the auspices of the newly formed Hunting Cocker Spaniel Club. The results were less than inspiring, with eight entries, none of whom were trained, but the enthusiasm of the owners persisted. With the assistance of several English judges the following year, the field trial of this club drew thirty-six entries, all of whom were American bred, with the exception of those running in a special international stake.

Cocker trials grew steadily in size and popularity, with several field trial clubs forming during the 1930s throughout the country. The Hunting Cocker Spaniel Club changed its name to the Cocker Spaniel Field Trial Club of America in 1929. It survives today, but holds trials for Springers only.

Until 1938 English Cockers almost never placed in competition against the American Cockers, but this dearth of rank changed with the performance of Cinar's Soot, a black dog owned and handled by E. Roland Harriman. Soot won the Open All-Age stake at the Cocker Spaniel Field Trial Club of America trials in Verbank, New York. E. Roland Harriman was a member of the prestigious New York family that produced W. Averill Harriman, a governor of New York and

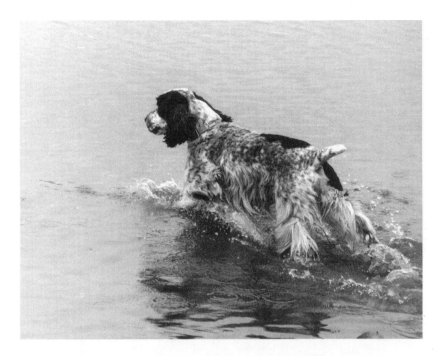

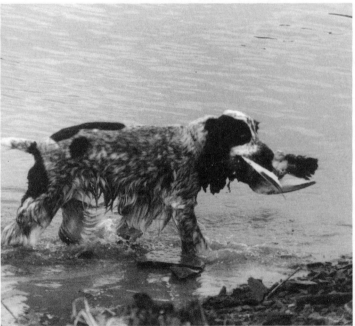

"Chauncey," owned by Emily McDermott, goes into the water for the bird and retrieves. "Chauncey" is formally known as Shaughnessy of Sprucerun, CDX, WDX, a blue roan and tan dog (Ch. Snowfrost of Sprucerun ex Sliversquill of Sprucerun).

82

world-acclaimed diplomat, and O. Carley Harriman, a well-known dog show judge. Roland, the youngest of the brothers, developed a line of working English Cockers bred from two Scottish imports in 1935. Dan of Cinar, a black dog bred to Merlin Mistletoe, a liver and white bitch, produced five field champions in four litters, among them the aforementioned Soot. The Harriman family estate was in Arden, New York. Part of the original estate became Harriman State Park, and on the remaining land retriever and spaniel trials were held and the kennels were maintained by Lionel Bond, Sr. The Cinar name was willed to Lionel Bond, who still raises an occasional litter of puppies descended from the original imports.

During World War II and in the years following, field trial activity declined dramatically. Only one English Cocker completed a dual championship when an Irish import, a solid liver dog, Arbury Squib from the West Coast, completed both his field and bench championships in 1941. The breed's second dual champion was Camino Boy, a black and white dog, also from the West, who completed his field title in 1947 and his bench title in 1950. Camino Boy was owned by H. C. (Dan) McGrew of Fortuna, California. He was the sire of three field champions and is behind many obedience and field titleists. To date, these two dogs are the only dual champions in the history of the breed.

During the 1950 there was a resurgence of interest in field trials, with several local clubs holding their own, and the beginning of the English Springer Spaniel Field Trial Association National Field Trial in 1953, which was open to all flushing spaniels. Dr. J. Eugene Dodson and Mr. "Dan" McGrew dominated the trial. Dodson's Wildacre Harum Scarum was the runner-up, and a Camino Boy daughter, Camino's Cheetah, won the championship.

National champions were scarce for several years until in 1958 another Camino dog, Fld. Ch. Camino's Red Rocket, won the title. Perhaps as interesting as this red dog's win was his ownership. He had been acquired shortly before the trial by actor Clark Gable, who apparently was a dedicated hunter and sportsman.

Interest waned again, and the last Cocker National Field Trial was held in 1962. Those fanciers who wanted to test their dogs in the field found few opportunities until the mid-1970s, when some English Cocker owners reactivated an agreement with the English Springer Field Trial Association to allow English Cockers to qualify for a Working Certificate under rules established by that body. In 1977 the first tests where English Cockers were run was the Maryland Sporting Dog

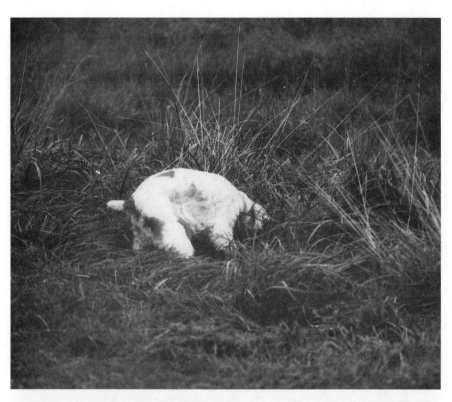

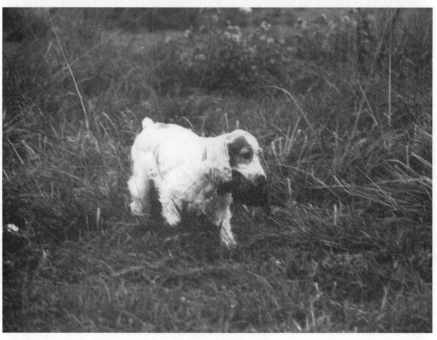

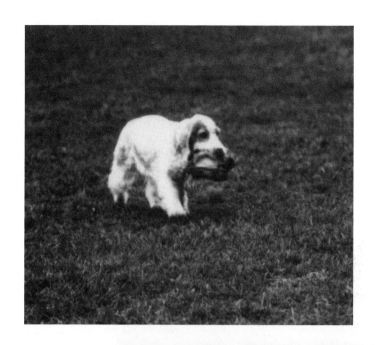

Carry-On Kerry Ceili, UD, TDX, WDX, an orange roan bitch (Foxfyre's Tarabrook Jasper ex Coltrim Cream Tea, CDX). "Ceili" locates, retrieves and presents the bird to hand.

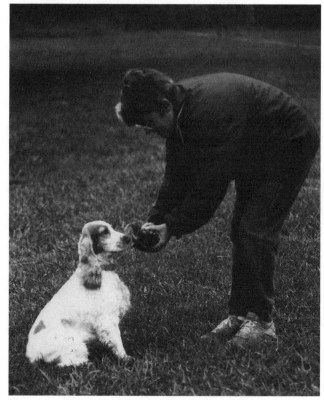

Association tests. Four dogs were entered, and three achieved their Working Certificates. They were Am. & Can. Ch. Merryborne Minstrel, WDX, owned by Deborah Mason; Am. & Can. Ch. Rose's Sherry Lenore, UDT, Can. UDTX, owned by Sue Rose; and Robert and Lorraine MacLennan's Ch. Mittenwald Gentian Andrew, who was awarded a WD.

English Cocker working tests have been very successful, and have replaced AKC-licensed Field Trials in most areas of the country. In the Northwest, however, the Pacific Northwest Spaniel Club and the Cascade English Cocker Spaniel Fanciers have held fun field trials in Spring and Fall, working toward AKC sanction.

In 1984 AKC instituted a new program of hunting tests for retrievers, and the following year issued guidelines for pointing breeds. Through the work of Deborah Mason, who was President of the ECSCA from 1986 to 1988, in conjunction with other spaniel clubs, notably the Welsh Springer Spaniel Club of America, the AKC approved rules for hunting tests for spaniels. It is almost certain that hunting tests will take the place of field trials for the English Cocker Spaniel in the foreseeable future.

INTRODUCING YOUR PUPPY TO THE FIELD

English Cockers are sporting dogs, and from the earliest days out of the whelping box the instinct to find things, to mark them by staring or pointing at them and to retrieve will become evident. There is nothing more delightful than to see a baby puppy, toddling on unsteady legs, spy a moth, an ant, even a shadow and stalk it, tail and rear end wagging furiously.

This instinct can be developed by praise and encouragement when the puppy finds and retrieves. Bringing back a ball or a stick which has been thrown will start the puppy on the right track to retrieving game.

When the puppy is about four months old you can begin training with a pheasant or a pigeon wing on the end of the fishing pole. This will imitate the flight of a live bird. The dog should be encouraged to find it and eventually to retrieve it. Associating the scent of a game bird with the desire to seek and retrieve is very important to the development of a good bird dog. A spaniel does not point game, but it should give some indication that it has found a bird before it flushes or retrieves it.

Basic obedience is important before taking the dog out into the fields to work on live birds. The dog must be responsive to the commands to fetch and bring, and respond to a call or whistle to come when it is called.

In order to give the dog the feel of a bird before actually taking it out into the field, you can attach bird wings to a retrieving bumper. Throw the bumper where the dog can see it and then send it out to fetch it. This can be done both on land and in the water.

Water retrieves are part of hunting and working tests for spaniels, and in order to be successful in this phase of the sport your puppy should be introduced early to the idea of swimming. Most English Cockers love the water and will take to it immediately. However, if you do not make the effort to get them into a lake or pond until they are older, they may be reluctant or afraid and will never be suitable waterfowl hunters.

You must be willing to take the dog into fields and hedgerows where pheasant, grouse and quail are to be found, so the dog becomes experienced at navigating rough ground, briars and bushes. Is this good for a show coat? No, it is not, but you and your dog will have such a good time that the loss of a few hairs will seem insignificant. To minimize the damage, you can put a heavy coat dressing on the feathers, which will enable you to brush out burrs with less difficulty.

Once you have introduced your puppy to the bird wings and have it retrieving to you at a short distance, you will be ready to venture out with the dog on a long line. You will need a friend to throw a bird, which has either been restrained or is already dead, ahead of the dog where the dog can mark the fall. Then you will send your dog to find the bird. Since you have the dog on a thirty-foot line, if it hesitates to bring the bird in, you can reel in the line while praising the dog for "achievement." Once the dog has the idea to watch where the bird falls you should begin shooting over the dog with blanks so it gets used to the sound of gunshot.

The next step is to have your accomplice throw several birds in different directions so the dog learns to "quarter the field," going from one hedgerow to another. Some dogs do this naturally, but others must be taught a proper hunting pattern.

After the dog has mastered these initial skills, it is time to go out to find live birds, either ones that have been put out ahead of time ("planted" birds), or native birds in their natural habitat. Coordinating the find, the flush (if the birds are live), and the retrieve after the birds have been shot takes patience and time. You will find that your English Cocker loves this instinctive game and that it is well worth the effort.

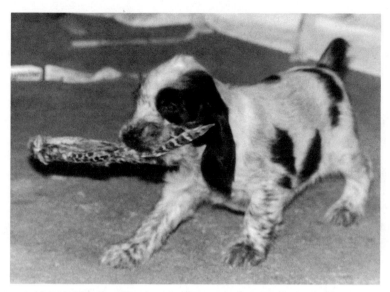
A promising youngster begins his training early. Owned by Betty Bathgate.

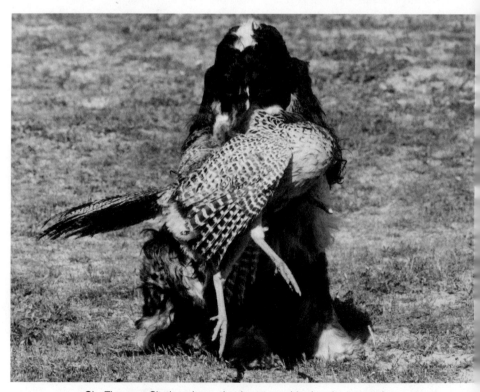
Ch. Timmara Citation shows that beauty and brains do go together.

There are many hunting clubs as well as local English Cocker Spaniel clubs throughout the country that can help you get your puppy started in the field. Since many people do not live where there is total access to fields and ponds, joining a group is one way to find the facilities and the friends to work with you and your puppy. Contact the American Kennel Club, 51 Madison Avenue, New York, NY 10010 for the name of the current officers of the English Cocker Spaniel Club of America. They can provide you with the name of the local club and members near you.

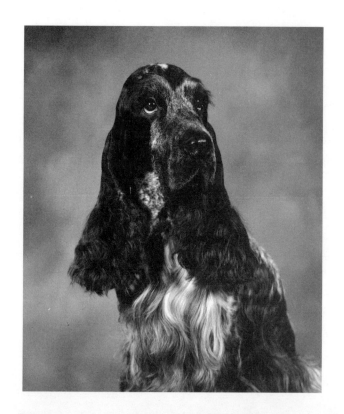

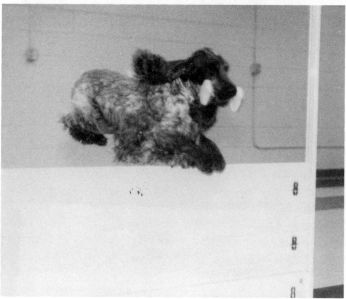

OTCh. Olde Spice Royal Commander (Ch. Carachelle Court Jester ex Ch. Cindione Andrea Christine, CD, WDX) at home and in the ring.

9

English Cockers in Obedience

ORGANIZED obedience trials in the United States were begun in 1936, and were largely dominated by working breeds, such as the German Shepherd Dog and the Doberman Pinscher. Standard Poodles did very well in obedience also, largely because of the impetus given to the program by its founders, Helene Whitehouse Walker and Blanche Saunders.

The first English Cocker to earn a CD was Basquaerie Buff King, a red dog bred and owned by Mr. and Mrs. Francis Crane. The Cranes were predominantly known for their Great Pyrenees, although they had a number of English Cockers during the 1930s and 1940s. The first champion English Cocker to win a degree was Ch. Blackmoor Beaconblaze of Giralda, CDX. He was also the first CDX English Cocker and the first dog of any breed to be awarded a perfect score, a feat he accomplished at the Greenwich Kennel Club show in June 1940.

The first two UD titles for English Cockers were achieved in 1953, when Captain's Roanokes' Falconer and Inky Pendant both won their titles.

The first UDT was Louise Shattuck's Kiwi's Carry-On Cricket in 1967. Louise's interest in obedience began in the 1940s and con-

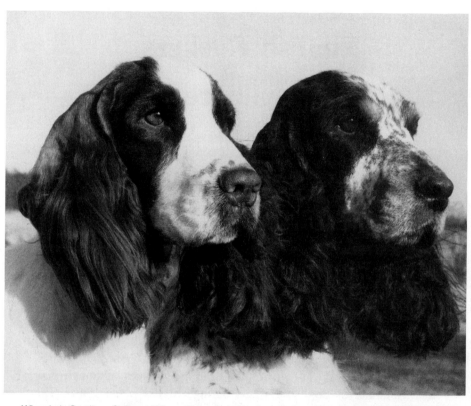

Wingslade Southern Colony, UDT, and Wingslade Southern Cause, CDX, TD, both owned by Cynthia Harrell.

tinues to this day. She has bred more English Cockers with obedience titles than any other person, fifty-nine and still counting!

The first English Cocker Champion UDT was Hiddenbrook's Jay Bee, bred by Mary Smith and owned by John and Mary Bonyai. He was a blue roan dog by Ch. Glengaddon Lucky Star ex Dunelm Priscilla. He completed his last title in 1970.

In 1973 Louise Shattuck's Carry-On Crispin of El Paca became a Champion UDT, as did Sue Rose's Sherry Lenore.

In 1978, obedience trials became part of the Engish Cocker Spaniel Club of America National Specialty shows and have remained a popular attraction at this prestigious event.

In 1980 the first Obedience Trial Champion was made. He was O.T.Ch. Brazos River Waco, UDT, WD, a blue roan dog bred by Suzanne Dillin and owned by Phillip Marr.

The 1980s showed an increase in obedience interest, with more English Cockers added to the roster of titleholders. Among them are Haywood and Cynthia Harrell's Delashire Journey South, UDTX, WDX; Wingslade Southern Colony, UDT; and Wingslade Southern Cause, CDX, TD. Southern Cause (Rebel) was Highest Scoring Dog in Trial at both the 1982 and 1984 ECSCA National Specialties.

Linda Klaer's Ch. Olde Spice Royal Commander, UD, is another top obedience contender, and one who competes successfully in both conformation and obedience.

The English Cockers are a versatile breed. Their happy, willing-to-please temperaments, combined with their keen noses and inquisitive natures, make them natural candidates for the active competition which both field and obedience tests provide. As we enter the 1990s they will continue to hold their own in these activities, and as the breed gains in popularity, obedience candidates will become more numerous.

INTRODUCING YOUR PUPPY TO OBEDIENCE

Obedience is basically manners. Anything you teach a young puppy can come under the heading of obedience. From the time it is born it is learning to adjust to its environment, and from the moment you bring a young puppy into your home, it will be influenced by what you teach it.

Housetraining, for instance, is a perfect example of obedience training. You will teach the puppy to eliminate in certain areas and

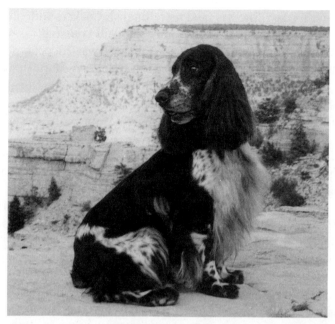

OTCh. Delashire Journey South, UD, TDX, WDX, blue roan dog (Delashire Domino ex Patbarossa Silver Lining).

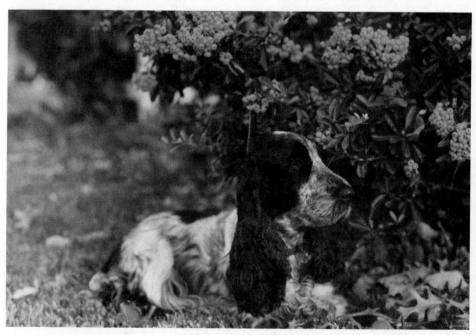

Ch. Carry-On Pogety Possum, CD, TD, WDX, blue roan bitch (Ch. Dunelm Smoke Signal of Wenloe ex Ch. Carry-On Rackety Coon, CDX, TD).

94

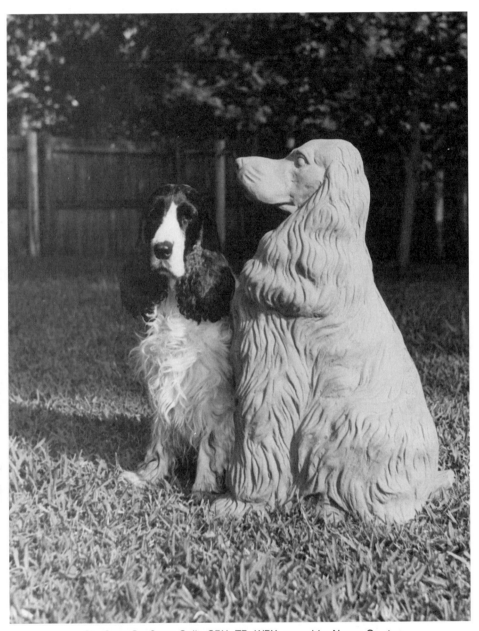

Ch. Carry-On Crazy Quilt, CDX, TD, WDX, owned by Nancy Overton.

not in others. By so doing, you are teaching it to be obedient to your wishes. When you teach it to walk on a lead, you are showing it how to stay with you, to follow or walk at your side without dragging you all over the street. These basic courtesies are all part of what eventually can be formal obedience training.

All puppies should learn basic obedience in order for them to be good companions and good neighbors. It is one of the responsibilities of owning an English Cocker to train it to be a good citizen.

We also talked about retrieving as being necessary for field work. It is also essential for any formal obedience or tracking.

The puppy can be taught to seek and find by playing the child's game of hide and seek. Start by "hiding" a person or an object within view and encouraging the puppy to find it. Every time the puppy does what is asked, give it lavish praise. *Keep the games short.* You can teach a puppy all the basic commands, such as "come," "sit," "lie down" and "fetch," when it is very young, about three or four months. Although it may not be steady all the time, when the time comes for formal obedience training, it will remember what you taught as basic manners.

Positive Reinforcement

All training with English Cockers must be done with positive reinforcement. That means lots of praise for doing it right. English Cockers have been called the "flower children" of Sporting dogs. They do not respond well to harsh handling. They are most anxious to please and will do anything for an encouraging word or a treat.

There are a few excellent obedience training books available that can guide you through the steps to training an obedience dog. For this breed, it is essential to choose an author whose training philosophy stresses the positive with praise and reward. Two such authors are Carol Benjamin and Job Michael Evans.

There are also dog obedience clubs that offer classes from novice to advanced, and will help you train your dog for formal obedience competition, if you so desire.

English Cockers are natural trackers, and tracking has become a popular pastime for many owners and their dogs. Other English Cocker owners can help you learn the ins and outs of tracking. Tracking clubs can also help, and provide the ground necessary to teach your dog to track. The American Kennel Club can provide you with the name of a local tracking club in your area.

OBEDIENCE TITLES AND COMPETITION

American Kennel Club competition is divided into several levels of difficulty. The Novice class is for dogs who are just beginning an obedience career. The exercises are relatively simple. Dogs must heel, both on and off lead, sit and stand for examination. As a class, they will sit and lie down for one and three minutes respectively. Upon completing three trials with scores of at least 170 and more than 50 percent of each exercise, the dog is awarded a Companion Dog (CD) certificate. You may then enter the next level, called Open. In this class the dog must perform all the Novice exercises, plus jumping and retrieving. When the dog has achieved the needed qualifying scores, a Companion Dog Excellent (CDX) degree is awarded by the AKC. The highest level of obedience is Utility. In this class the exercises are more difficult, including Scent Discrimination and a Signal (no voice) exercise. If your dog succeeds with passing grades in Utility, you have a UD titleholder.

One other level of achievement is possible. That is an OTCH (Obedience Trial Champion), a title earned only after the dog has attained a UD. To become one a dog must win one hundred points by repeatedly taking first or second place in Open B or Utility classes according to regulations established by the AKC.

The best way to decide if obedience competition is for you is to go to a few obedience trials and watch. If you decide that it looks like fun, then you must go through obedience training courses.

A word of caution about obedience courses and trainers. Given the nature of the English Cocker, you'll want to go to one whose instructor teaches by using praise and not punishment. You should attend a few classes and watch the teaching techniques. Don't rush in to plunk your money down until you're sure you like the instructor, the class members and the atmosphere. Then, if you decide to enroll, don't assume that your dog's fate is out of your hands. If you don't like what transpires after a couple of sessions, don't stay. It is not likely that your money will be refunded; however, your dog's personality and well-being are at stake.

YOU AND YOUR DOG—PARTNERS IN TRAINING

Some English Cockers have a great affinity for obedience. Their merry dispositions and eager attitudes make them quick and willing pupils. An obedient dog also makes a better and more trustworthy companion.

Obedience training with English Cockers requires about a half hour of dedicated time each day. It can be divided into two periods, morning and evening, in which you and your dog work together without interruption. This should be done whether or not you attend organized training classes

Obedience must be taught step by step so that the dog understands exactly what is expected at all times. The advantage of attending obedience classes is that the instructor teaches you how to teach your dog. Then, when you practice at home, you will be following the correct procedures.

You should practice your lessons at a time when you are not in a great rush, and are able to concentrate in a focused manner. Do not practice when you are angry or feeling particularly impatient. The dog will sense your mood and will not work well. Do not use obedience training as an excuse to vent hostility toward your boss, your spouse or your kids. In the process you will ruin your English Cocker, possibly forever.

To begin your obedience training you will need a six-foot-long leather lead with a snap clasp and a nylon choke collar. If you are doing both obedience and conformation work, use different collars and leads and different commands for each activity. The dog will soon learn to differentiate and act according to the circumstances.

Heel

The first lesson usually is learning to heel. The object is to teach your dog to walk beside you, paying attention to you without straying, following a scent or dragging behind.

Attach the lead to the collar on the dead ring (that is the ring which does not pull up on the choke) and roll it up in your right hand. Step forward with your dog on the left side, at the same time saying, "Buster, heel!" in a firm tone. The dog's natural inclination will be to look at you and follow along. If your dog does this, give lots of praise and keep going. Maintain a good pace and do not adjust your stride to the dog. Your dog must learn to follow your lead. The minute "Buster" begins to stray from your side, give a jerk on the lead and repeat the command. Do not drag the dog along, but encourage it with words and little jerks on the lead. As soon as you have Buster going along well for two or three minutes, praise with a "Good dog," and

98

Ch. Edgewood Play With Fire, CD (Ch. Reklawholm Firebird ex Ch. Graecroft Calliope) executes a good return following the **retrieve on the flat**.

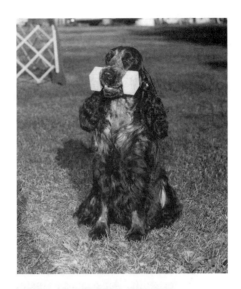

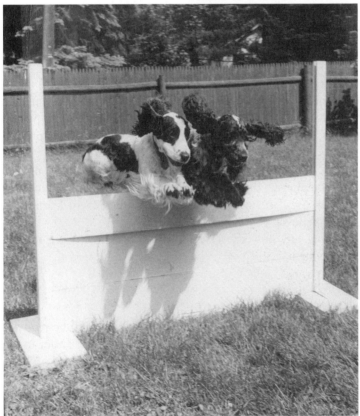

Carry-On Kelpie, UDT, and Ch. Carry-On Kipper Cottontail, UDT, clearing the **high jump**.

some special word that you will use consistently to signal the end of the exercise. It can be "okay," "all done" or "cheese and crackers." The dog won't understand the precise words, but will recognize by the tone of your voice and by your actions that the lesson is over.

Keep the lessons brief and always end on a positive note. Do not end the lesson unless the dog has done what you have asked, if only for a fleeting moment.

Sit

The next lesson you will learn is to teach the dog to sit. You may have already taught this if, as a puppy, the dog sat for a treat. If so, you can easily carry this over to your obedience lessons. If not, place your left hand under the dog's hindquarters and with your right hand pull up on the collar. Say "Buster, sit!" as you slide your left hand underneath. As soon as Buster sits, give lots of praise. Repeat this procedure several times, and then give the command without guidance. If the dog obeys, give lots of praise and quit the lesson. If not, go back to guiding Buster into a sitting position until he gets the idea.

A word of caution about commands. Give them *once* in a clear, firm voice. There is no need to shout. A dog's hearing is better than yours, but constant nagging will cause the dog to turn off and pay no attention until you start yelling, and that defeats the whole purpose of obedience.

Once heeling and sitting are mastered, you are ready to put the two lessons together. "Buster, heel!" you say, and after you have gone several steps, "Buster, sit!" Eventually Buster will learn to sit at your side whenever you stop.

In teaching any new exercise, you must break it down into its simplest components.

Stay

Once Buster has learned to heel and to sit, you will be ready to teach the stay (in place) on command. You will instruct Buster to sit, then walk one or two steps away, turn and face the dog and give the command "Stay!" without attaching any name to it. Your dog will undoubtedly get up, at which instant you return Buster to the original spot and repeat the command. When Buster stays put for one minute, end the exercise. Gradually you will be able to extend and vary the length of time that the dog must sit in one spot.

Down

After sitting comes lying down, an exercise most dogs like until they are commanded to do it! Put your dog in a sitting position, lift the front legs with your right hand, pull gently forward on the collar with your left hand and command "Down!" giving the dog no choice but to hit the floor. If Buster pops up, repeat the exercise until he stays lying down. Make sure it is a comfortable position. Once the dog really understands down, give Buster the command "Stay!" and keep the "down-stay" position for at least two minutes before giving a release.

The "down" exercise is very important for several reasons. You may want the dog to stay comfortably in one spot during your dinner hour, or while you are juggling packages at the car door. The "down" command can save lives, too. A dog ready to cross the street will not run into traffic if commanded to lie down. This command at a distance, however, is a far more advanced exercise than the beginners' class.

Putting a dog on a "down" or on a "long down" and requiring it to stay in one spot for as long as thirty minutes is an exercise in dominance. Any dog lying down on command is being put in a subservient position. For most English Cockers this is never a problem. They are not naturally dominant or aggressive dogs, but some animals like to be the boss of the household. This is not permissible under any circumstances in any human-dog relationship. One way to tell a dog that you are the boss is to enforce the "long down." You can do this while you are reading the paper or watching TV at night. You can do it while you are fixing Buster's supper or getting dressed to go out. The important thing is that you insist the dog stay down until you give the release word. This exercise need not be done every day. Once or twice a week is usually enough.

Come

The most difficult exercise and the one which most dog owners want above all is the "come." How often one hears the tale, "My dog won't come when called." Dogs are clever; they know when you can catch them and when they're out of reach.

The only way to have a dog who comes to you each and every time no matter what the temptations to escape is conditioning. From puppyhood you clap your hands to call "Buster, come!" in your most cheerful voice. Whether puppy or adult dog coming for a biscuit, the words must always be associated with pleasure. Lavish praise, treats, whatever the dog likes best must be the reward for coming. It is

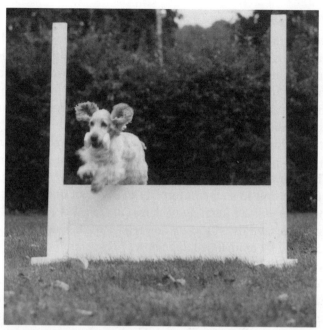

Retrieve over the high jump performed by Ch. Mistral Apricot Brandy, CDX, orange roan dog (Ch. Ashgrove Apache ex Mistral Apres Vu).

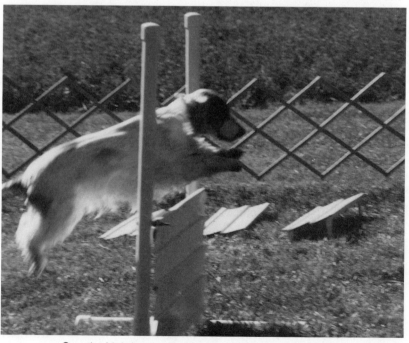

Over the **high jump** sails Carry-On Kerry Ceili, UDTX, WDX.

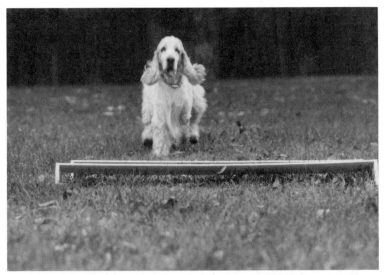
Ch. Mistral Apricot Brandy, CDX, takes the **broad jump**.

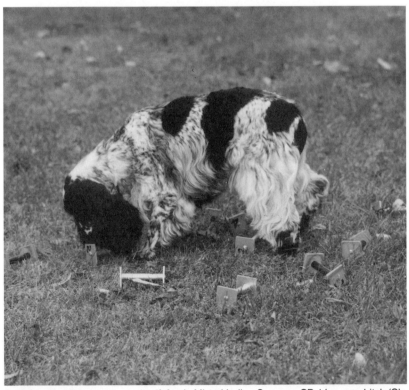
Searching for the correct **scent articles** is Mistral Indian Summer, CD, blue roan bitch (Ch. Barnhide Vision of Mistral, CD, ex Mistral Zircon).

essential to keep the dog in control all the time it is learning the command. It can be done on a long line, which you reel in as you call, or in a fenced area where Buster cannot escape. Your dog must never have the opportunity to disobey while you are teaching the command to come.

Never, ever call a dog to you in order to punish it for some other transgression. If you want to show the dog the sofa it has just ripped to shreds, go and get the dog and bring it to the scene of the crime.

Never, ever punish a dog who has come back to you, even if it shows up twenty agonizing minutes later. Your dog will associate the punishment with coming to you and you can kiss that command good-bye.

With these basic commands—"heel," "sit," "stay," "down" and "come"—you can build all the other obedience exercises you will find in regular competition. You can teach your dog to fetch the dumbbell, to jump over high and broad jumps, to retrieve gloves and to stand for examination.

Some of these exercises can be very useful in the show ring, too. Teaching your dog to trot along on a loose lead looks very much better than to have the dog choked up on a chain. The "stand for examination" exercise can be used to stack the dog. Tell it to "stay" and step back, giving the judge an unobstructed and very impressive view of your dog.

Altogether, obedience training serves multiple purposes, not the least of which is to forge a closer bond between you and your English Cocker.

TRACKING WITH YOUR ENGLISH COCKER

AKC Obedience Regulations state that "the purpose of a tracking test is to demonstrate the dog's ability to recognize and follow human scent and to use this skill in the service of mankind."

Tracking Dog (TD) and Tracking Dog Excellent (TDX) are two additional titles which AKC bestows and for which the versatile English Cocker eminently qualifies. The sport of tracking is challenging, fun, and greatly rewarding. It demonstrates, more than any other AKC degree, the close relationship and trust that exist between human and dog.

Tracking is a sport in which the human is totally dependent upon a canine partner to find the "quarry" at the end of a predetermined, but unknown to dog and handler, path or "track." The person must be able to "read" the dog, that is to be able to ascertain by the motions and mannerisms of the dog the correct direction of the track and trust the dog enough to follow its lead. Many a tracking title has been lost because of the handler's inability to trust the dog's scenting ability.

One tracking story that illustrates this bond involves an elderly gentleman and his dog. The spectators at this event were treated to a chilling demonstration by dog and handler. They began their track, proceeded to the second flag and without hesitation began their journey. Slowly the dog led the way, with the handler following at the end of the tracking line. At the turns, the dog cast for the correct direction in a methodical manner. Upon completing an almost perfect track, the dog found the dropped article and merrily took it to the owner. The spectators cheered. What made this particular team so beautiful to watch? The man was blind.

Tracking, in brief, involves the following:

1. Plotting the track on paper and in the actual field where the track will be run. This is done by the tracking judge on the day before a trial. The track must be between 440 and 500 yards long and must include at least two right-angle turns. The track is outlined by flags, which are set at the beginning and at various points and turns along the path.

2. On the morning of the trial a tracklayer will walk the track to impart an unknown human scent to the track. The tracklayer will leave the first two flags in place, but will remove the remaining flags as he or she walks the track. At the end of the track an article will be dropped, such as a glove. The tracklayer will then proceed in a straight line off the course.

3. After the track has aged approximately one hour,* the dog and handler will be brought to the first flag. Working in a harness with at least a twenty-foot lead, the dog will be urged by the handler to follow the track. The dog should lean into the harness and pull the handler to the second flag. There the dog must ascertain the direction of the track and lead the handler in that direction. The track is completed when the dog finds the dropped article and signifies that find, usually by picking up the article. If it is evident that a dog is not working and is taking too much time on a track, especially at a turn,

---

*AKC regulations state that for the TD test the track must not be less than one half hour or more than two hours old.

or if a dog wanders too far off the track, upon the concurrence of both tracking judges, a whistle is blown and the dog will be called off the track. Standing alone with your dog in the middle of a big field and hearing that whistle blow is the most dreaded sound in the sport.

The Tracking Dog Excellent (TDX) title is a more complicated version of tracking. Two tracks are laid, with one intersecting the other at different places. The track is at least 800 to 1,000 yards, and must contain at least three right-angle turns. A typical track contains at least five but not more than seven turns. The track can contain obstacles, such as a fence, stream or road, or it may go through fields and woods. Four articles are dropped along the path of the track, which must then be designated as found by the tracking dog. Only one flag is used to mark the beginning of the track, thus allowing at least 180 degrees for the direction of the start of the track. The dog must follow one track and not be diverted by the decoy track. The track must be at least three hours old and not more than four.

English Cockers, being Sporting dogs, can easily be led astray as they track. The warm scent of a covey of quail is enough to interrupt the concentration of the most competent tracker. However, English Cockers, being a breed of dogs that are really attuned to their human friends' desires, can quickly be brought back to their challenging task.

Training English Cockers for tracking requires:

1. A tracking harness and a long lead (twenty to forty feet).
2. Open fields (baseball or football fields will do for training purposes).
3. A tracking companion or support group, such as a local tracking or obedience club or an English Cocker club with members who track.

Begin with a short, straight track, with your accomplice putting a glove where the dog can see it. Encourage the dog to find the glove, by leading you to it. Gradually you will increase the distance that the tracklayer goes, until the dog is attuned enough to go several hundred feet. Then you can begin tracking a turn, adding to the distance according to the amount of concentration the dog brings to the task.

Titleholders

In the years 1986 through 1988, thirty-eight English Cockers acquired their TD degrees and three received their TDX degrees. These

106

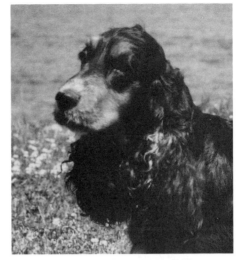

Gordon Hill Tartan Tri Me, UD.

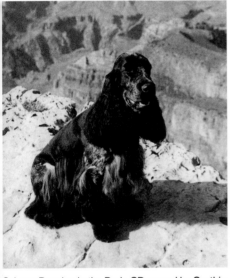

Sojourn Dancing in the Dark, CD, owned by Cynthia Harrell.

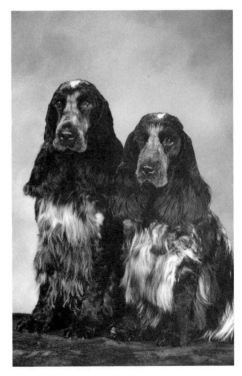

Can. Ch. Dundee's Moonlite Dancein, CDX, and Am. & Can. Ch. Malagold Moonlite Fantasy, UD.

dogs are found everywhere in the United States, although there are pockets of tracking activity in several areas. The northwestern United States, with the Cascade English Cocker Club, boasts many tracking English Cockers, including Ch. Kvammes Astral, bred and owned by Marlin and Lorrie Kvamme. Several of Carol Richter's Topsham English Cockers have acquired tracking degrees, and Beth McKinney's Paganhill dogs have also proved to be good trackers.

On the East Coast, most particularly in Massachusetts, one name is synonymous with tracking—Louise Shattuck. Louise can be considered a tracking trailblazer for the breed. She has been involved in it for over forty years, and to date has put sixteen TDs on her English Cockers. Kiwi's Carry-on Cricket, UDT, was Louise's first English Cocker to acquire a TD, in 1967. Louise finds the breed to be highly motivated, a quality that is essential for a good tracking dog.

Emily McDermott with her bitch, Carry-On Ceili, UDT, WDX, is another devotee of tracking, as well as field work for her English Cockers.

Cynthia and Haywood Harrell, who have called many parts of the United States home, have put many TD degrees on English Cockers, including their great obedience dog OTCH. Ch. Delashire Journey South, UDTX, WDX.

The Michigan area has also produced many good tracking English Cockers, including Sue Rose's great Ch. Rose's Sherry Lenore, WDX, Am. & Can. UDT, Can. TDX.

Texas fanciers have also taken tracking to their hearts.

Many Canadian English Cockers have acquired TD titles, including Can. & Am. Ch. Ranzfel Newsflash, bred and owned by Virginia Lyne. The Merrynook Kennels of Livia Whittall has produced many fine tracking dogs, including the first two English Cockers to earn TDX titles, Merrynook Marsh Marigold and Merrynook Saucy Sue.

10

Early Breeders

$\mathbf{A}$MONG THE EARLY FANCIERS of English Cockers in the United States, a few stand out, some of whom are active to this day.

Most important was **Geraldine Rockefeller Dodge**, who, married to M. Hartley Dodge, is credited with bringing the English Cocker into its own. Mrs. Dodge was a remarkable woman, by any measure. Blessed with intelligence, exquisite taste, a love of dogs and horses and ample funds to pursue her interests, she was able to contribute in lasting ways, not only to the dog fancy, but to animal welfare.

Giralda Farms, where Mrs. Dodge maintained a kennel of up to 150 dogs of many breeds, was situated in rural Morris County in New Jersey. It was a showplace, which she opened to the public once a year on the occasion of the Morris and Essex dog show. That show, which was last held in 1957, has never been equalled in elegance or splendor. Every detail bore the stamp of Mrs. Dodge's attention. Trophies were of sterling silver. Butlers in uniform served luncheon under huge tents for all the exhibitors and judges. The grounds were impeccable, ringed by specimen trees and flower gardens.

By the 1950s, however, the show had become so large that Mrs. Dodge felt she could not control it as she wished and so it was discontinued. She turned her energies into the establishment of an animal shelter, St. Hubert's Giralda, and set aside an area on her estate for

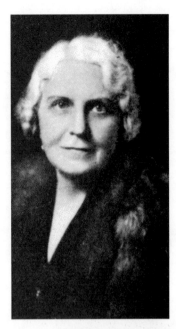

Geraldine Rockefeller Dodge
(Mrs. M. Hartley Dodge).

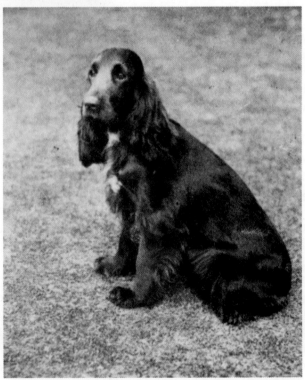

Ch. Blackmoor Bronze Model of Giralda, liver bitch (Ch. Blackmoor
Beacon of Giralda ex Ainslee Zoe).

110

it. When she died, the shelter was endowed with land and money to build and maintain a first-class facility. St. Hubert's has become a model humane shelter, but it is more than that. Adjacent to the shelter was built an art gallery and library to house the most precious of Mrs. Dodge's vast art collection. A historical record of the English Cocker is contained in that library, along with many paintings of her dogs, including Ch. Blackmoor Beacon of Giralda and many of his descendants.

Louise Platt, Mrs. Collier Platt, has been involved with the English Cocker since the 1930s. From her home in Syosset, New York, have come some of the great solid Cockers, many descended from her original import bitch, Ch. Coral of Zorro. Mrs. Platt's most famous ambassador for the breed, however, was a spritely red imported dog, Ch. Buff Tip of Broomleaf. Buffy was whelped in 1974 and brought to the United States as a puppy. He enjoyed an illustrious career, handled by Laddie Carswell, who, with his daughter, Candy, has managed Mrs. Platt's kennels for the past thirty years. The Platts' **Merrythought** kennels have not produced many dogs in recent years, and with the death of Collier Platt in late 1988, activity was further reduced. The Platts, however, were instrumental in causing the English Cocker to be recognized as a breed in the 1940s.

Anne Rogers Clark, one of the nation's top professional handlers in her youth and now a world-esteemed judge, started her career in dogs literally from birth. Her mother, Olga Rogers, was an astute and enterprising dog breeder and seller. Olga became interested in English Cockers in the 1930s, and the **Surrey** prefix began with the offspring of several dogs which she imported for clients. Among the most important of these were Chartwell Boots, Mixed Posey of Miklebuffe and Merryworth Mariner. They are found in many modern pedigrees, and although Anne no longer breeds English Cockers, she is still considered an authority on the breed. Many Surrey dogs are found in important pedigrees today. Perhaps one of the most famous litters bred by her was the "Surrey Blue Hen" litter in 1972 containing Surrey Blue Stone and Surrey Blue Jean. Blue Stone was purchased by Ruth Cooper, and although he finished his championship handily, he was most valuable as a stud, siring thirty-three champions. Surrey Blue Jean was purchased by E. Irving Eldredge for his wife, Ann, as a foundation bitch. She produced eight champions and was the start of Maidavale English Cockers.

Another early fancier was **Ethelwyn Harrison**, who acquired her first English Cocker, Capricious Vic of Ware, from a breeder in Ohio

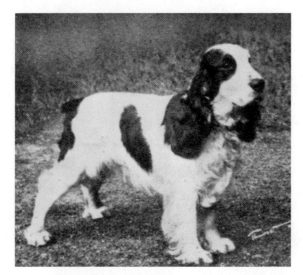

Eng. Ch. Colinwood Cowboy, blue roan dog (Blackmoor Brand ex Colinwood Cigarette).

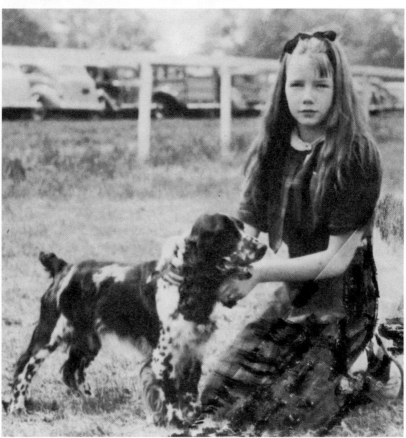

Anne Hone Rogers (Clark) at age nine, with Merryworth Mariner.

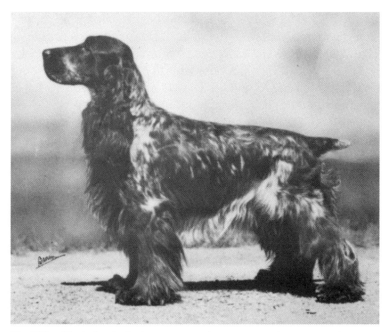

Ch. Shikar Wyn's Sentinel, blue roan dog (Ch. Lanehead Distinction of Giralda ex Ch. Blackmoor Bronze Model of Giralda).

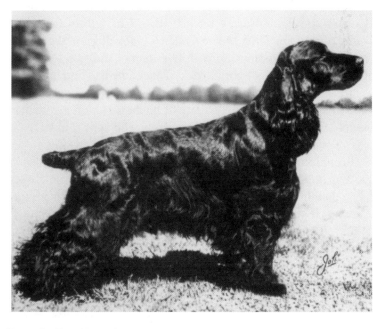

Ch. Surrey On Time Morse Code, black dog (Ch. Surrey Sea lark ex Surrey Merry Sinner).

in about 1935. She registered her kennel name, **Shikar Wyn**, in 1937 and began to import dogs from England. During the next decade, under the guidance of Geraldine Dodge, she brought in several Blackmoor dogs. She bought Ch. Blackmoor Bronze Model of Giralda from Mrs. Dodge and bred her to another Giralda dog, imported Ch. Lanehead Distinction of Giralda. This produced Ch. Shikar Wyn's Sentinel, whelped in 1941. She continued to breed and show her dogs, at one time accommodating as many as a hundred at her farm in Ohio. By the time she had retired from active breeding and showing, more than fifty Shikar Wyn champions had been recorded, many of whom appear in today's pedigrees. Ethelwyn Harrison died in 1983.

In 1947 **Maurie and Seymour Prager** bought their first English Cocker from a breeder in New York City, where they were living at the time. Prager's On Time Susie was soon joined by another bitch, Surrey Merry Sinner, a black, bred by Olga Rogers. Their first litters were bred soon after, and the **On Time** kennels was launched. Within a few years the Pragers moved to Middle Valley, New Jersey, where they proceeded to develop a strong line in the ninety-plus litters they bred over forty years. Maurie was the breeder and mainstay of the kennel, and when she died in 1975 the kennel was sold and Seymour moved to a city apartment. He is still active in English Cocker club affairs.

One of their most famous and influential dogs was whelped in 1948 from the black Surrey bitch bred to Ch. Surrey Sea Lark. He was Ch. Surrey On Time Morse Code. A black dog, on the small side, he finished his championship with five majors and two Best of Breed wins. "Johnny" was a hybrid black. That is, he had one line of solids, through his dam, with the rest particolors in his background, and he produced all colors bred to a variety of bitches. He left eighteen champion get with many particolor descendants who appear in today's pedigrees. Some solids appear through the Merrythought line.

From Johnny's first litter, in 1950, bred to On Time Winter Moon, came the important liver roan bitch, Ch. On Time Susie Belle. She produced eight champions, the most important of which were the Best in Show–winning blue roan bitch Ch. On Time Amanda; Ch. On Time Deborah, a black and white ticked; Ch. On Time Rosalie Sue, a blue roan; and Ch. On Time Susette, a blue roan.

The offspring of these bitches were behind many of the modern kennels, among them Woodlea-Dicroft, Kenobo, Wingslade, Somerset and Soho.

The Johnny/Winter Moon breeding was repeated in 1953, pro-

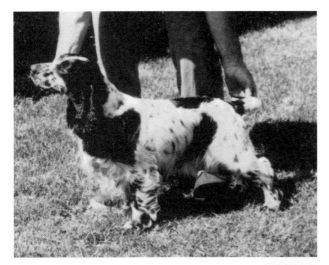

Ch. On Time Deborah, black and white ticked bitch (Ch. Springbank Ace of Giralda ex Ch. On Time Susie Belle).

Ch. Free Chase Pumpkin Coach, liver roan dog (Ch. Barnabus of Heidesta ex Ch. Silvermine Cinderella), handled by Jane Kamp (Forsyth).

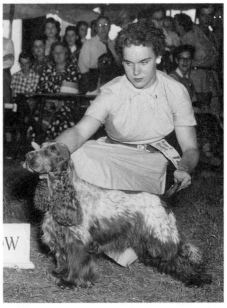

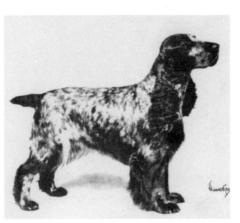

Ch. Surrey Eventide, blue roan bitch (Mikado of Ware ex Ch. Blue Cornflower of Edgeley).

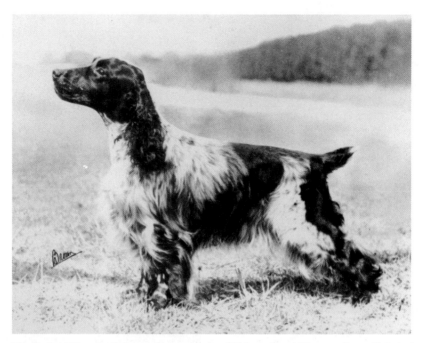

Ch. Squirrel Run Confederate, blue roan dog (Wideawake of Ware ex Sweet Rebel of Fasseroe of Ware).

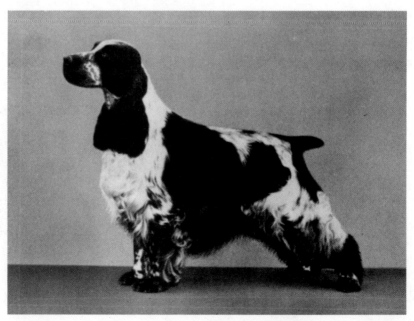

Ch. Glengladdon Lucky Star, blue roan dog (Valstar Lucklena Minstrel ex Glengladdon Blue Diana).

116

ducing Ch. On Time Richard, a blue roan dog who is behind everything with the Graecroft and the Wyncastle names. Richard also sired Ch. On Time Albert, National Specialty winner in 1958, Ch. Soho Bluejay, CDX, and Ch. Soho Prodigal Son, both of these being woven throughout the pedigrees of Soho, and through Ch. Soho Beguiling behind many of those with the Paganhill name.

Maurie and Seymour Prager's dedication to the breed, their love of the English Cocker and their careful breeding program, based largely on linebreeding, with an occasional judicious outcross, has profoundly influenced the course of the English Cocker Spaniel both in the United States and in England. On Time bloodlines are still felt today, though Seymour himself is no longer actively breeding dogs.

Jane Kamp Forsyth, liker her contemporary Anne Rogers Clark, grew up with dogs. She entered the show ring at the age of ten and has never left it. At twenty she became a professional handler and in partnership with Mr. and Mrs. George Pusey founded **Grayarlin** Kennels. Over the years Grayarlin moved to Connecticut, where, in association with her husband, Bob, it became one of the foremost professional operations of its kind in the country.

Jane handled many English Cockers throughout her career, and her advice enabled many kennels, including Grayarlin, to prosper. Some of the kennels with which she was associated were Heidesta, Free Chase, Elblac and Joyanne.

No discussion of important kennels of the past would be complete without mention of **Squirrel Run**, the establishment of **Mr. and Mrs. Hallock duPont** in Wilmington, Delaware. The name was registered with the American Kennel Club in 1933, and the first of the Squirrel Run English Cockers was Lucky Maid of Ware, imported in 1932. English Cockers, however, did not play a sustaining role at Squirrel Run until after World War II, when Hallock and Virginia acquired several dogs from the renowned Mr. Lloyd. Most of the English Cockers produced at Squirrel Run over the next thirty years were the results of imports, most of them from Herbert Lloyd. Few puppies were sold and few Squirrel Run dogs were offered at public stud, but occasionally one was brought out. One such was Ch. Squirrel Run Confederate, an American-bred dog from British imported stock. He was whelped in 1953, made quite a name for himself in a short time in the show ring and then was sent to England, where he was shown by Mr. Lloyd and used at stud. He returned to the States in 1956, where several of his get finished. Through them his name appears in modern pedigrees. Virginia duPont died in 1984, her husband having predeceased her by many years.

Abracadabra, the kennel name belonging to **Mary Elizabeth Dyer deGaris**, was registered in 1946, but "Babs" deGaris imported English Cockers from Europe in the 1930s. After World War II, Babs became acquainted with Olga and Anne Rogers, whose advice she followed in establishing her breeding program. She has continued to breed English Cockers of various lines, and has bred more than forty champions. In 1989 a black and tan, Abracadabra Kingby Clement (Ch. Abracadabra Corry ex Kingbys Mynerva), won Best of Winners at the American Spaniel Club show in New Jersey.

Birchwyn, the name of the kennel established by **Mary Livesey, M.D.**, with the guidance and partnership of Ethelwyn Harrison, has produced some seventy champions over the past thirty years. Dr. Mary first became interested in English Cockers toward the end of the Second World War. She acquired her first Shikar Wyn bitches in the late 1940s and in 1952 teamed up with Ethelwyn Harrison, who from then on supervised the breeding program. Dr. Mary became very interested in health problems of the English Cocker and has established the Birchwyn Fund to provide money for research into genetic problems that afflict the breed.

During the 1950s, several breeders entered the ranks of English Cocker fanciers. Many are active today and can be found in this book in the chapter on English Cockers of today. Among these are **Jane and Arthur Ferguson**, whose **Dunelm** English Cockers have had an enduring influence on the breed.

Roland and Patsy Rickford founded **Rick N Pat's** kennels in the early 1950s. They are still active today, with more than thirty champions to their credit.

As we move into the 1960s, two dogs stand out as being influential in the development of the breed. One was Ch. Glengaddon Lucky Star, bred and owned by Dr. Donaldson Beale Cooper, and the other was the English dog Ch. Courtdale Flag Lieutenant.

Lucky Star was the top English Cocker for three years. He was a stylish, balanced dog who sired twenty champions. His most important get were Ch. Dunelm Stardust and Ch. Dunelm Dictator. Through these two he is found in nearly all modern particolor pedigrees.

English Show Ch. Courtdale Flag Lieutenant was a blue roan dog, whelped in January 1963. He finished his championship at the age of two, but as a sire he made a lasting mark both in England and the United States. Five of his get became American champions, and his name is found in many pedigrees today.

118

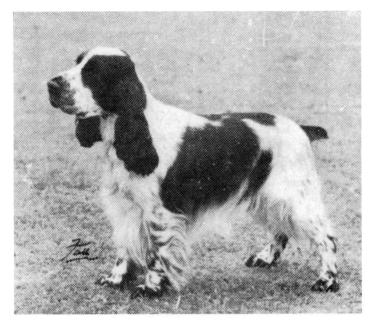

Eng. Ch. Courtdale Flag Lieutenant, blue roan dog (Courtdale Colinwood Seahhawk ex Courtdale Kinkellbridge Gina).

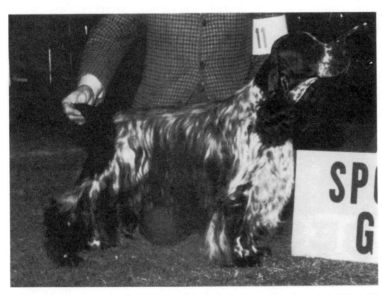

Ch. Ancram's Simon, blue roan dog (Ch. Ancram's Oliver ex Ch. Courtdale China Mink).

Soho English Cockers were born in the early 1960s, although **Lynn Clark**, their founder, began to own them in the mid-1950s. Her first show-quality English Cocker was Quarto K Alert's Son, from the Salt Lake City kennels of Laura Clark (no relation). He was a black dog that she bred to Ch. On Time Deborah, a bitch leased from the Pragers. About the same time she was able to acquire the litter sister to Alert's Son, a red bitch, Quarto K Titian Blonde. She bred this bitch to Ch. On Time Bertram, a liver roan. From these two litters and the addition of Ch. On Time Richard came the foundation of all the Soho dogs. During the next twenty-five years Lynn and Harry Clark bred more than a hundred champions, and the Soho influence is found in many lines throughout the country. Lynn died in 1988, having been ill for several years, and left a legacy of wisdom. She was a witty and creative person, who used her knowledge of anatomy and genetics to mold a line of English Cockers that will have lasting impact on the breed for generations to come.

Joyce Scott-Paine founded the **Ancram** Kennels in Ancramdale, New York, in the late 1950s with an orange roan import, Ricmour Crystal Dawn. She was bred twice, and her offspring were combined with two dogs imported in 1965, Ch. Courtdale China Mink, a blue roan bitch, and Ch. Courtdale Buccaneer, a black and white dog. Over the ensuing years, almost forty champions have borne the Ancram prefix, but none more important than Ch. Ancram's Simon. Simon was whelped in June 1965, out of China Mink sired by Ch. Ancram's Oliver. During his career Simon won eighteen Bests in Show, a record standing to this day. He sired thirty-six champions during his illustrious career.

The history of any breed is only as good as the breeders who foster it. The English Cocker Spaniel is fortunate in having a small enough group of breeders to be able to maintain type and consistency throughout the years. The breed has also benefited from a continuing interchange of blood stock between the United States and England. From the earliest days to the present, dogs cross the Atlantic, although today, because of strict quarantine laws in Great Britain, fewer are imported there than are sent to our shores. We continue to profit from a gene pool that has gone back more than a hundred years and that continues to influence our dogs today.

11

Breeders of Today and Tomorrow

A BREED is as strong as the people who support it. They are those dedicated breeders who love the English Cocker and strive to perpetuate and improve upon its endearing qualities. In this chapter are some of those breeders who have built upon the firm foundations of past sires and dams, and who will be the pillars of the breed in the years to come.

George and Mary Ann Alston, Maryland: Fieldstone

Mary Ann and George Alston have made a lifetime commitment to dogs and the sport of dogs. Although several breeds call Fieldstone home, the English Cocker holds a special place and meaning in their lives.

Among the most special of the Fieldstone Cockers was Ch. Fieldstone Maesgwyn Katydid. This beautiful blue roan bitch, sired by Ch. Graecroft Star Duster, became a multi–Best in Show winner and a top-ranked English Cocker.

Ch. Fieldstone Maesgwyn Katrina, co-owned with Marie Thompson, has proven her worth as a dam. Some of her champion offspring include Fieldstone Bachelor Button, Fieldstone Black-Eyed Susan and Fieldstone Blue Cadet.

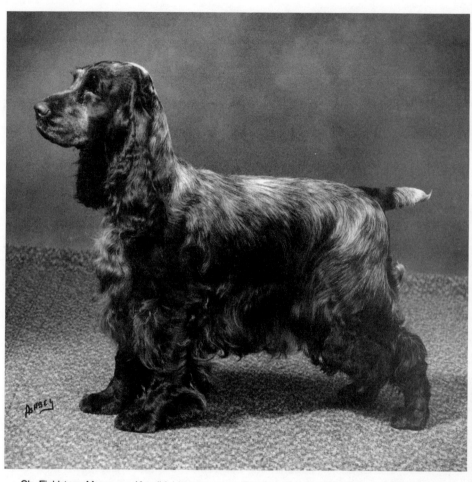

Ch. Fieldstone Maesgwyn Katydid, blue roan bitch (Ch. Graecroft Star Duster ex Dunelm Maesgwyn Moonshadow).   *John L. Ashbey*

Also taking up residence at Fieldstone is the blue roan dog Ch. Kvammes Hollywood, TD, bred by Marlin and Lorrie Kvamme. Woody was an Award of Merit winner at the 1987 National Specialty and is proving his worth as a sire.

Ch. Edgewood Play with Fire, CD, TD—"Ernie," as he is affectionately called—also holds a special place at Fieldstone and with his many fans. Ernie, who was the winner of the first English Cocker Futurity, is the sire of many champions, all of whom possess his indomitable spirit and merry temperament.

Marjorie Auster, New York: Southwind

Marjorie has owned English Cockers since 1950, but has been actively breeding and showing since her retirement as a teacher in 1977. She currently owns four champion bitches, notable among them Ch. Druid Little Miss Muffet, bred by Dana Davis and owned by Marjorie, who made breed history by completing her championship in fifty hours with three five-point majors. Quite an accomplishment! Muffet is the dam of five champions to date.

Other residents of Southwind include Ch. Mourning Dove Merry Too, Ch. Southwind Misty Mourning and Ch. Southwind Kelpie. Mourning Dove is the dam of four champions; Misty Mourning has two champions to her credit.

Mary Jane Barnes, Minnesota: Moonlite

Although Mary Jane's involvement with English Cockers spans a short time, she has accumulated some notable accomplishments.

One of her first accomplishments goes by the name of Am. & Can. Ch. Malagold Moonlite Fantasy, UD, Can. CD. Bred by Meridith Guy and Mary Hopkins, she was Mary Jane's introduction to the breed. In 1986 "Ashley," as she is called, ranked as one of the top English Cockers in obedience with an average score of 197.5. In 1988 she completed her Utility Degree (UD) in three consecutive shows with a first-, third- and fourth-place win in the Utility ring. Ashley was bred once to Ch. Reklawholm Rockbeat and is currently in training for the field.

Another accomplishment of Mary Jane's is Can. Ch. Dundee's Moonlite Dancein, CDX ("Bentley"). Bred by Jane Bond and Sharon Collins, Bentley completed his Canadian championship in one weekend. He is also pointed in the United States with multiple Best of

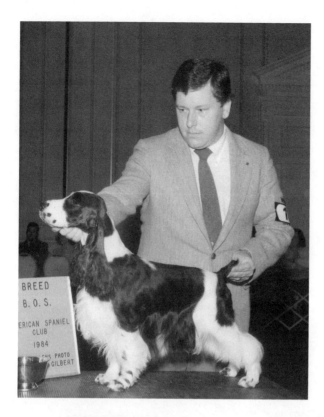

Ch. Druid Little Miss Muffet, black and white bitch (Ch. Kenobo Confetti ex Ch. Graecroft Bewitching).

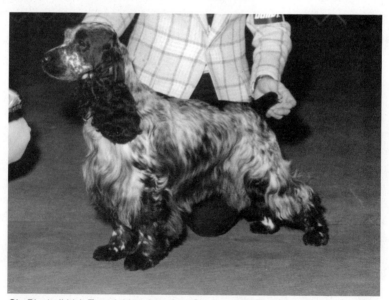

Ch. Bluebell Irish Tweed, blue roan dog (Ch. Amawalk Cottleston Concorde ex Ch. Bluebell Caryn). *William P. Gilbert*

124

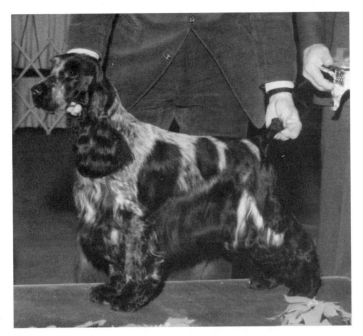

Ch. Perrocay Curzon Corregidor, blue roan dog (Ch. Kenobo Capricorn ex Ch. Cottleston Chaos). *John L. Ashbey*

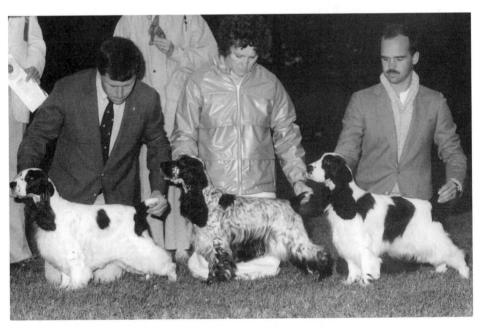

Left to right: Ch. Log Tavern Phara Sunshine, black and white bitch; Ch. Log Tavern Autumn Skylark, blue roan bitch; and Ch. Log Tavern Sassy Suzy Q, black and white bitch.

125

Breed wins to his credit. His work in the obedience ring is also impressive, as he was the top-ranked English Cocker in 1987 with an average score of 198.3.

Betty Batchelder, New York: Bluebell

Betty acquired her first English Cocker from the Pragers in 1965. With encouragement and instruction from the Pragers, Betty showed her and was hooked on the sport. Next came On Time Vivian's Bridey, a lovely orange roan, who with the help of Richard Bauer had a brief and successful trip to her championship.

Hoping to combine the soundness and substance of On Time with the elegance and showmanship of Ch. Dunelm Galaxy, Betty bred Bridey to Galaxy and achieved her goal. From that first litter came Ch. Bluebell Boomerang, a liver roan bitch and a delightful showgirl who achieved championship status with four major wins. From a repeat breeding of Bridey to Galaxy came another showy liver roan bitch, Ch. Bluebell Irish Mist.

In 1974, with a firm resolve to continue her line breeding to Galaxy, Betty bred Irish Mist to Ch. Surrey Blue Stone, a Galaxy grandson. From that litter came Ch. Bluebell Caryn, a light-blue roan bitch co-owned with Mary and Greg Wysocki. She in turn was bred to Ch. Amawalk Cottleston Concorde and produced Ch. Bluebell Irish Tweed. Shown by Richard Bauer on a limited basis, Irish Tweed had an impressive show career and became the top winning English Cocker in 1980. He is the sire of multiple champions. Another breeding of Caryn, to Ch. Maidavale Firethorne, resulted in four champions.

To date, Betty has bred eight litters and has bred and/or owned eighteen champions, including four Group-placing dogs and several obedience titled dogs.

Betty Bathgate, Pennsylvania: Log Tavern

Betty's love of the breed spans eighteen years and began with the very lucky acquisition of the bitch Phara The Divine Miss M (Ch. Kenobo Capricorn ex Ch. Kenobo Happiness Is). This bitch, "Deva," was bred to Ch. Roundelay Rival and produced Ch. Log Tavern Phara Sunshine, a Group winner and outstanding producer. "Sunny" in turn produced Ch. Log Tavern Stage Door Debut, the 1983 English Cocker National Specialty Best of Breed winner, owned by Randy Feather and Martin Sellers; Ch. Log Tavern Kabree Love, the 1983 Specialty

Sweepstakes winner; Ch. Log Tavern Song Sung Blue; Ch. Log Tavern Autumn Skylark; and Ch. Log Tavern Sassy Suzy Q.

Deva's second breeding to Ch. Roundelay Rival produced the two outstanding workers Ch. Log Tavern Fancy Pants, CD, WDX, and Log Tavern Lad of Meadowrue, CD, WDX. Lad is well known for his enthusiasm, skill and desire in the field.

The Log Tavern breeding program is based on the use of dogs that are sound both physically and mentally, dogs that win in the breed ring and work with enthusiasm and success in the field and in obedience.

Richard L. Bauer, New York: Curzon

Richard Bauer has been showing English Cockers for thirty years. He is a top professional handler whose most famous English Cocker charge was Ch. Dunelm Galaxy, whom he showed for Ruth Cooper. Galaxy remained with Richard throughout his life, and it was Richard who guided the dog's great career as a show dog and top stud dog.

His first Best in Show English Cocker was Ch. Squirrel Run Burgomaster, owned by Hallock and Virginia duPont, in 1960. Richard was, at that time, an assistant to Anne Hone Rogers (later Anne Rogers Clark).

He began breeding English Cockers in 1980 with a Galaxy daughter out of Ch. Surrey Blue Witch, Ch. Cottleston Chaos, a blue roan bred by Ruth Cooper and originally owned by Ed Jenner from Wisconsin. His partner in the ownership and breeding aspect has been Scott Proctor (Perrocay), whose first English Cocker was Am. & Can. Ch. Kenobo Blue Astro, CDX, Can. CD.

Chaos, bred to Ch. Kenobo Capricorn, was the dam of the multiple Group-winning brothers, Ch. Perrocay Curzon Corregidor and Ch. Perrocay Curzon Cozumel. Corregidor remained with Scott and Richard. Cozumel went to Texas, where he is owned by Valerie Johnson, Rita McKissack and Terri Burrows.

The most titled dog owned by Scott, Richard and Harry Proctor is American, Canadian, Bermudian, Bahamian, Puerto Rican, Las Americas Ch. Amawalk Perrocay Qeqertag, a blue roan dog bred by Betty Ganung. "Pacman" finished his championship at ten months, was Best of Breed at the AKC Centennial Show in 1984 and is a Best in Show winner with over a hundred Group placements. He is the sire of six champions to date. He was sired by Ch. Kenobo Confetti out of Ch. Amawalk's Katrina.

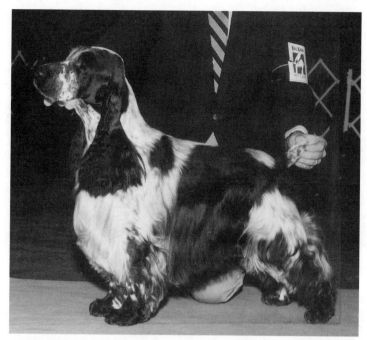

Ch. Amawalk Perrocay Qeqertag, blue roan dog (Ch. Kenobo Confetti ex Ch. Amawalk Katrina).   *John L. Ashbey*

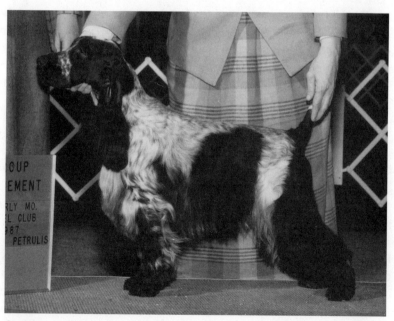

Ch. Jaybriar's Simon, blue roan dog (Ch. Reklawholm Rockbeat ex Ch. Parade Pegeen).
Don Petrulis

128

Chaos was bred to Qeqertag in co-ownership with George Britto to produce Ch. Perrocay Curzon Cherry Grove and Ch. Perrocay Curzon FIP. Cherry Grove was bred to Ch. Fleet St. Fidelio, CD, to produce the current generation of Bauer-Proctor dogs, one of whom, Perrocay Curzon Sanibel, was the Best Bred by Exhibitor at the American Spaniel Club show in 1988.

Judy Monroe Beebe, Iowa: Jaybriar

Judy acquired her first English Cocker in 1978, finished her first champion in 1980 and bred her first litter in 1981. Since then Jaybriar has bred thirteen champions. Jaybriar is very much a family affair, with Judy's son Paul and daughter Lyn both being very successful in Junior Showmanship.

That first champion, Ch. Touchwood Tidings, CD, WD, is the dam of three champions, including Ch. Jaybriar's Zither, CDX, Jaybriar's first homebred champion.

Jaybriar's most famous English Cocker is Ch. Parade Pegeen, CDX, a blue roan bitch bred by Kathryn Kinowski and Tracy Lazarus. Pegeen has proved to be a winner in all phases of the sport. She has been a top ranking obedience dog, a multiple breed winner and, most importantly, a top producer with ten champions to her credit and many more pointed offspring. One of Pegeen's most notable sons is the Group-winning Ch. Jaybriar's Simon, owned by Kathy and Terrance Zimmerman.

Pegeen's daughter Ch. Jaybriar's Sonnet, co-owned with Diane Gibson, finished her championship at the 1986 Jubilee National from the 9-12 puppy class. Pegeen, not to be outdone by her baby daughter, won the Veteran Bitch class at this National and was named Best Veteran by beating the Veteran Dog. Judy's daughter, Lyn, capped this very successful show by winning Best Junior Handler with Pegeen.

Patricia Beresford, Connecticut: Patchwork

After seeing many English Cockers in different situations and liking the breed enormously, Pat expressed a wish to Mary Ann Alston of Fieldstone Kennels to own one. Mary Ann had recently acquired a young bitch from Tom Bradley's Luftnase Kennels. And so Luftnase's Blue Becomes Me, or "Misty," as she was affectionately called, came to live with the Dachshunds at Patchwork and more than fulfilled the desire for "several Engies."

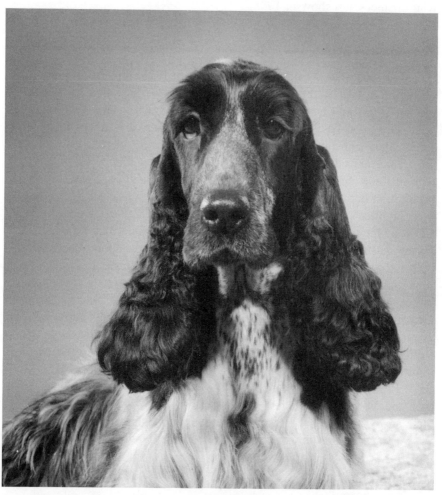

Luftnase's Blue Becomes Me, blue roan bitch (Ch. Surrey Blue Stone ex Maple Lawn Winter Rose).
John L. Ashbey

130

With Mary Ann Alston as the breeder of record, Misty was bred to Ch. Kenobo Constellation and produced Ch. Fieldstone Silver Dream and Am. & Can. Ch. Fieldstone Sterling Silver.

Misty was then put in co-ownership with Mary Ann Alston and bred to Ch. Graecroft Star Duster. From this litter came Ch. Fieldstone Blu Sky, who sired the Best in Show dog Ch. Buettner's Black Jack. An outstanding bitch from this breeding was Ch. Patchwork's F'ldstone Moody Blu, who was Best Puppy in Sweepstakes at the 1977 English Cocker National Specialty.

A second breeding to Star Duster produced Ch. Patchwork's Second-Hand Rose, who became the foundation for Ann Perry's Ballywheel Kennels. Rose in turn produced Ch. Ballywheel Blue Chip and Ch. Ballywheel Blackthorne.

Bred a final time to Ch. Kenobo Rabbit of Nadou, Misty produced a rainbow of colors: a blue roan, a black and white, a blue roan and tan and an orange roan. Several of this rainbow coalition went on to acquire championships. Misty was an ECSCA Top Producer in both 1978 and 1979.

From a show career point of view the most noteworthy dog bred by Patchwork was Am. & Can. Ch. Patchwork's Just In Time, a blue roan dog. His career record was 6 Bests in Show, 80 Group placements, and 130 Bests of Breed in Canada alone. He was owned by Richard Rouchefort at the time.

Lynette Boyd, Florida: Diplomat

Lynette's story begins with her daughter Eve, who at the age of twelve years handled their first show dog to his championship. This dog, Ch. Glenmora Diplomat in Brass, has proven to be an excellent sire. One of his sons, Ch. Rustlin Puttin on the Ritz, UDT, has been a top-ranked obedience dog.

Ch. Highcliffe Heaven Sent became the foundation for the Diplomat solid-color Cockers. She produced three champions from her first litter sired by Am. & Can. Ch. Rustlin Gallant MacDuff: Ch. Rustlin Dauntless Diplomat, who finished at eighteen months of age with a Best of Breed win; Ch. Diplomat So Much Velvet, who finished at ten months; and Ch. Diplomat's Jack Daniels, who acquired his championship in grand style with five major wins.

Ch. Sunspan Bonfire, a lovely orange roan, has become the foundation for the Diplomat roans. She has produced Ch. Diplomat's Country Girl.

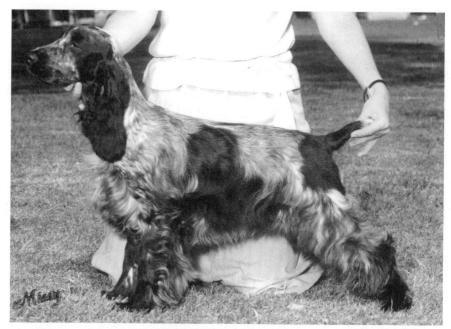

Ch. Kabree Silver Spark, blue roan dog (Ch. Olde Spice Crusader ex Ch. Log Tavern Kabree Love).
Missy Yuhl

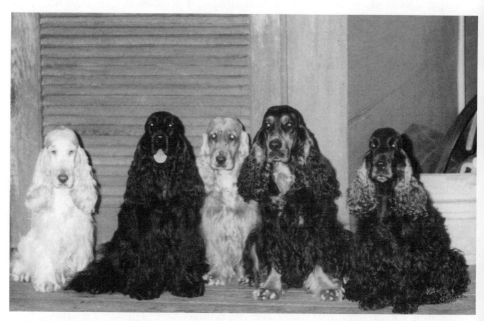

Left to right: Ch. Sunspan Bonfire, orange roan bitch; Ch. Diplomat Jack Daniels, black dog; Ch. Highcliffe Heaven Sent, red bitch; Ch. Glenmora Diplomat in Brass, black and tan dog; and Glenmora Midnight Melanie, CD, black bitch.

Mr. and Mrs. E. M. and Kerri Brangers, Ontario, Canada: Carnaby

Carnaby English Cockers began in 1968, with the purchase of their foundation bitch, Can. Ch. Brandmoor's Flair. She was an orange roan puppy chosen from a litter bred by Dr. Hart and Dr. Edith Steinbeck of Unionville, Ontario. Her ancestry was from the two old English kennels, Colinwood and Of Ware.

Carnaby is a small hobby kennel whose aim is to produce English Cockers pretty enough for the show ring, yet stable and healthy as family pets.

Carnaby produced Can. Ch. Carnaby Calico, who was Reserve Winners bitch over a record entry at the 1983 English Cocker Spaniel Club of America National Specialty, held in Ravenna, Ohio. Their most successful combination was the mating of Am. & Can. Ch. Olde Spice Crusader and Am. & Can. Ch. Carnaby Capricious. This produced Can. Ch. Carnaby Quintessence, one of their recent winners. Two of her littermates also finished in Canada, and a repeat breeding has produced four more Canadian champions.

Kathleen Buchanan and John Moore, California: Kabree

In 1978 Kathleen Buchanan purchased her first English Cocker, a lovely blue roan dog bred by Marlin and Lorrie Kvamme, by the name of Kvamme's Classic Cowboy. Cowboy became the first champion at the Kabree household, completely owner handled by Kathleen.

The foundation of Kabree is Ch. Log Tavern Kabree Love, a black and white bitch sired by Ch. Kenobo Capricorn and out of Ch. Log Tavern Phara Sunshine. Kabree Love won Best in Sweepstakes at the English Cocker Spaniel Club of America National Specialty in 1983.

Ch. Kabree Silver Spark, a son of Kabree Love and sired by Ch. Olde Spice Crusader, is probably the most famous Kabree production to date. Silver Spark finished his championship with four majors in one month of showing. Shown as a special on a limited basis, he garnered several Best of Breed wins, a Group I win and several other Group placements.

Nancy and Darrell Buettner, Wisconsin: Darcy

Dixie's Midnight Magic was Darrell and Nancy's first introduction to English Cockers and the world of dog showing. Dixie soon became a champion and they were hooked!

133

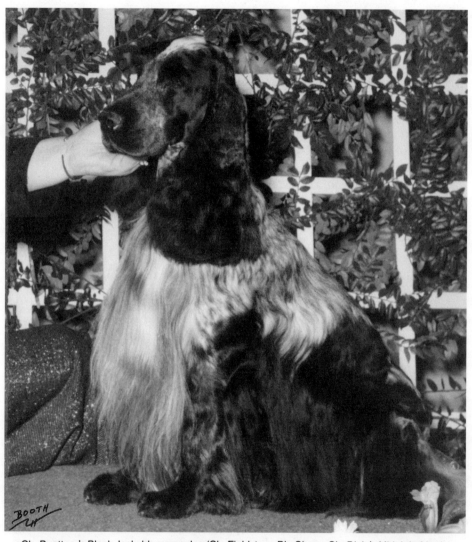

Ch. Buettner's Black Jack, blue roan dog (Ch. Fieldstone Blu Sky ex Ch. Dixie's Midnight Magic).
Booth Photo

Dixie was then bred to Ch. Fieldstone Blu Sky, and from that first litter of three came Ch. Buettner's Black Jack, who streaked to his championship at eight and a half months of age, winning a Best of Breed in the process. He was the youngest English Cocker to finish that year. Jack went on to a very successful show career that included five Bests in Show and twenty Group I wins. Jack was piloted through his show career by Connie Gerstner.

Jack also proved to be successful as a stud. From a litter out of Ch. Canterbury's Oreo of Malagold came a stud fee puppy that was to become Ch. Darcy's JJ of Malagold. JJ's impressive career includes four Best in Show wins and eleven Group I's. He was the number one English Cocker in 1986.

JJ in turn has also produced very nicely. Among his offspring are Am. & Can. Ch. Malagold Moonlight Fantasy, UD, Can. CD, who is owned by Mary Jane Barnes, and Stardust Morse Code, owned by Nancy Malichar, who has a Group placement from the Puppy class.

Terri and Ron Burrows, Texas: Idyll

Idyll English Cockers began in 1978 with the acquisition of a light blue roan male who would become Ch. Winsonem Idyll Admiral (Ch. Applewyn Angus ex Ch. Birchwyn Burnt Smoke). He was specialed only occasionally and was a mutiple Best of Breed winner and sire of numerous champion offspring.

Ch. Perrocay Curzon Cozumel, co-owned with Rita McKissack and Valerie Johnson (Essentia), is now an important part of Idyll. Timmy finished in the top ten rankings of English Cockers for 1985, 1986 and 1987. Always owner handled, he has been a consistent breed and Group winner. Timmy has multiple major-pointed puppies and at least one champion son to his credit. Timmy was bred by Scott Proctor and Richard Bauer.

Debbie and Bill Campbell, California: Sandcastle

Debbie purchased her first English Cocker from Jodelle Burke of Wyncastle Kennels in 1980. His name was Wyncastle's Cherlock Holmes, and he completed his championship easily at thirteen months of age. Since then Debbie has bred, owned or co-owned fifteen champions.

Ch. Wyncastle Lookin At You Kid, a dog owned by Debbie, became a Group winner and sired many champion offspring. One of these champion offspring, Ch. Glenwood Sandcastle Deju Vu, had the honor of becoming the top English Cocker in the country in 1987. His impressive show career included four Bests in Show, and fourteen Group I wins. He holds the record of being the youngest English Cocker to win a Best in Show, a feat he accomplished when he was fourteen months of age!

Janina Cirillo, Massachusetts: Cabaret

Janina Cirillo has been a breeder, owner and exhibitor of English Cockers for twelve years. Although Jan breeds and exhibits her dogs on a limited basis, her kennel, Cabaret, is home to some lovely, top winning English Cockers.

Ch. Cedarhurst Jonathan Seagull, bred by Marta W. Smith, is a multiple Best of Breed winner, a multiple Group placer and, most importantly, has proven to be a top producing sire through 1987.

Jonathan has sired Ch. Cabaret Country Robin, a multiple breed and Group placer, who went Winners Bitch and Best of Opposite Sex at the prestigious American Spaniel Club show in 1985.

Cabaret Jenny Wren, also sired by Jonathan, repeated the thrill for Jan in 1986 when she also went Winners Bitch at the American Spaniel Club show.

Ch. Dunelm Alice Blue Gown, co-owned with Jane Ferguson, and Ch. Cabaret Snow Pixie also call Cabaret home.

Muriel Clement, Connecticut: Gordon Hill

When Muriel looks at her dogs she sees black . . . and tan. Beautiful black and tan Gordon Setters and English Cockers reside at Gordon Hill Kennels. Muriel's love of Gordon Setters spans over forty years; her love for and involvement with English Cockers is more recent, beginning in 1971.

Muriel's first English Cocker was Ch. Topjoy's Sad 'N' Saucy, CD, an English import of solid color breeding. Because of a scarcity of black and tan males in the eastern United States, Saucy's first two mates were blacks that were sure to produce the black and tan color. In 1977 she was bred to Ch. Abracadabra Lasso and produced a black and tan litter. From that litter came Gordon Hill Sad 'N' Saucy Too, CD, TD. She in turn was bred to five black and tan dogs. Of Saucy Too's twenty-three black and tan puppies, five have been bred and produced more black and tans, and eight have competed at various

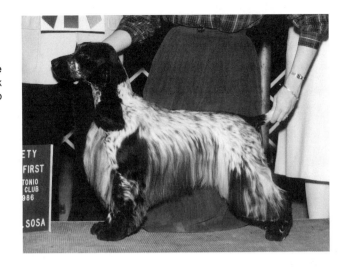

Ch. Darcy's JJ of Malagold, blue roan dog (Ch. Buettner's Black Jack ex Ch. Canterbury's Oreo of Malagold).

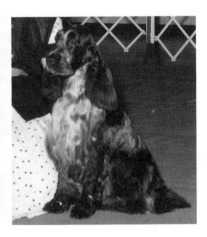

Ch. Perrocay Curzon Cozumel, blue roan dog (Ch. Kenobo Capricorn ex Ch. Cottleston Chaos). *Booth Photo*

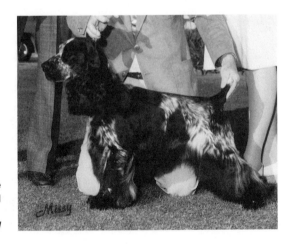

Ch. Glenwood Sandcastle Deja Vu, blue roan dog (Ch. Wyncastle Lookin At You Kid ex Ch. Glenwood's Starr of Redwitch).
Missy Yuhl

137

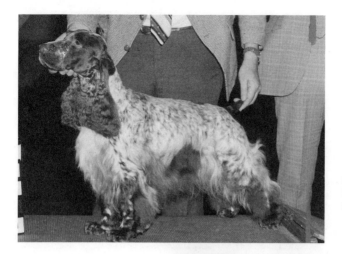

Ch. T-Flite's Major Dundee, CD, liver roan dog (Ch. Surrey Blue Stone ex Vari's Champagne).

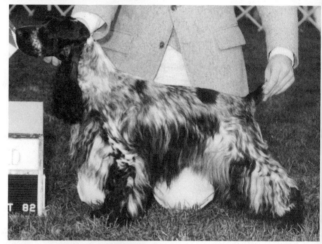

Ch. Aberglen My Fair Lady, blue roan bitch (Ch. Reklawholm Firebird ex Ch. Woodlea-Dicroft Pennyroyal).

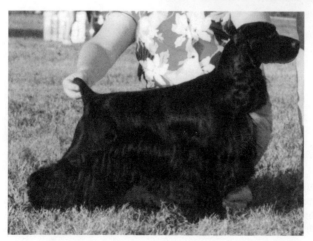

Ch. Canterbury's Fireside Shadow, black bitch (Ch. Briarpatch Magic Marker ex Canterbury's Chimney Sweep).
Paulette J. Brodbeck

138

AKC events. The versatility of these little black and tans is shown in Saucy Too's children and grandchildren: Gordon Hill TarTan Tiffany, CDX, TD, and Gordon Hill TarTan Tri Me, UD.

Sharon Collins, Illinois: Dundee

Sharon's involvement with English Cockers began in a big way with the purchase of what was to be a family pet from Michael Bagley. This dog, Ch. T-Flite Major Dundee, CD, a liver roan, became a multiple Best in Show winner.

From Sharon's interest and involvement with Major Dundee's show career came her interest in breeding English Cockers. Her Ch. Springfield Top Page O'Dundee ("Bandit") sired four champions. Sharon purchased two bitch puppies, Ch. Springfield Ladybug O'Dundee, a "Bandit" daughter, and Ch. Stoney Creek Kiapolo O'Dundee. Both bitches have produced champion and Group-placing offspring.

Ladybug, bred to Ch. Southwind's Braemar's Classic, produced two American champions and a top winning obedience dog, Can. Ch. Dundee's Moonlite Domain, CDX. He has received both the American and the Canadian Dog World awards.

James Covey, New York: Aberglen

Aberglen English Cockers came about as the result of the friendship and decision to "join forces" between Jim Covey and Rochelle Schwarz Lafer.

Aberschan English Cockers started in 1969 with the purchase of Ancram's Jessica. In 1971 Jessie was bred to Ch. Dunelm Galaxy, producing the first two homebred champions for Aberschan: Ch. Aberschan Jeremiah and Ch. Aberschan Tuppence of York. Tuppence was then bred to Ch. Kenobo Capricorn.

Shelglen Kennels, in the meantime, had purchased and finished the light-blue roan and tan bitch, Ch. Windswept's Elizabeth, bred by Jeanne Brecht.

At this point, Shelglen and Aberschan joined together with the co-ownership of Ch. Aberschan Flair of Shelglen, a bitch resulting from the Capricorn/Tuppence breeding. A lovely bitch, she did much for Jim and Rochelle and produced, among others, Can. Ch. Shelglen's Catherine of Ahoy.

The Capricorn/Tuppence breeding produced a total of four champions, making Tuppence one of the top producing bitches for that year.

One of the most notable offspring from that litter was Ch. Aberschan Reginald, a very flashy light-blue roan dog. Reggie, owned by Jeanne Brecht, completed his championship at one year of age. A multiple Group winner, he also garnered a Best of Breed win at the 1977 National Specialty and the 1978 American Spaniel Club show. Reggie is the sire of nineteen champions, including a Best in Show winner and two top producers.

Ch. Woodlea-Dicroft Pennyroyal, a Reggie daughter, came to Aberglen as a result of a tip from friend David Flanagan, who had seen her litter and thought she looked promising. This striking black and white bitch won her first major from the Puppy classes, then went on to the 1978 English Cocker National in California, where she garnered Best in Sweepstakes. She finished that same weekend with two five-point major wins.

In 1981 Penny was bred to Ch. Reklawholm Firebird and produced Ch. Aberglen My Fair Lady, co-owned with James Zabawa, who became a third, very active partner in Aberglen. Lady finished her title with four majors and three Best of Breed wins. From Lady's first litter, by Ch. Edgewood Liberty Valence, came Ch. Aberglen Grizabella. From her second litter, sired by Ch. Edgewood Fan-Tan, have come some promising youngsters, including Aberglen Mickey Finn.

Aberglen operates on a small scale, keeping only a handful of dogs and breeding approximately one litter a year.

JoAnn Larsen Davis, Michigan: Canterbury

The foundation of JoAnn Larsen Davis's Canterbury Kennels was built on two bitches acquired from Mike and Rita Atkins of Vari Kennels. The first was Am. & Can. Ch. Vari's Pajama Party, a black and white bitch; and the second was Am. & Can. Ch. Vari's Fascination, a blue roan.

Pajama Party ("P.J.") was bred three times and produced five champions. One breeding of P.J., a black and white particolor, to Ch. Birchwyn Bentley, a solid black dog, produced the future line for Canterbury solid English Cockers. This litter produced two champions: Ch. Canterbury's Headmaster, owned by Mary Francis DeLamerens, and a black bitch, Ch. Canterbury's Tea 'N' Crumpets, who achieved her championship at the age of ten months. Crumpet was then bred to Ch. Abracadabra Rufus De Nita, owned by Karen Prickett. This breeding produced two black females, Ch. Canterbury Chimney Soot and Ch. Canterbury's Chimney Sweep.

Ch. Canterbury's Chimney Sweep was a top producer, with eight champions to her credit. Sweeper's most prestigious and influential offspring is Am. & Can. Ch. Canterbury's Fireside Shadow ("Mona"). Mona took her first major and Best of Breed on the day she was six months old. She went on to complete her championship in seven shows, before she was ten months old. Her illustrious show career includes both an American and Canadian Best in Show, and a Best of Opposite Sex and Award of Merit at past English Cocker Nationals.

Mona is also a top producer. Her first litter, sired by Am. & Can. Ch. Wittersham's Emblem, produced Ch. Canterbury's Enchantment, a Best in Sweepstakes winner at the 1986 English Cocker Club of America's Jubilee National Specialty. Her second litter, sired by Ch. Hobbithill Ashwood Hi Class, has produced three champions: Ch. Canterbury's Class Act, a red male owned by Susan D. Fiore; Am. & Can. Ch. Canterbury's Entertainment, a black bitch owned by JoAnn; and Ch. Canterbury's Governess, a black bitch owned by Helen Nothelfer and co-owned by JoAnn. All three of these dogs finished before two years of age with many Specialty wins.

JoAnn's second foundation bitch, Am. & Can. Ch. Vari's Fascination ("Cindy"), also finished very quickly and became a Group winner. However, Cindy's best efforts were in the whelping box. She produced fourteen champions from a total of twenty-two puppies whelped, a truly amazing percentage. Her progeny have been winners at the American Spaniel Club, Westminster Kennel Club and various Specialties.

Currently residing at Canterbury is a red male, Am. & Can. Ch. Lochranza Touching Wood, who was imported from Lochranza Kennels in England. "Jodi," as he is called, is co-owned with Myra Main and Susan Fiore.

To date Canterbury has bred forty champions.

Gail and Mark Dehayes, Georgia: Hobbithill

Mark and Gail Dehayes joined the ranks of English Cocker lovers in 1976 with the purchase of a blue roan bitch from Beth McKinney. This bitch became Ch. Paganhill Jasmine On Parade.

The second bitch to join Hobbithill was Gaybrook Amber of Hobbithill, a red bitch bred by Gaynell Griffin in Canada. Amber completed her championship with four majors, completely owner handled by Gail. Amber may be a breed champion, but her real championship abilities are as a brood bitch. Bred three times to Ch. Hubbestad

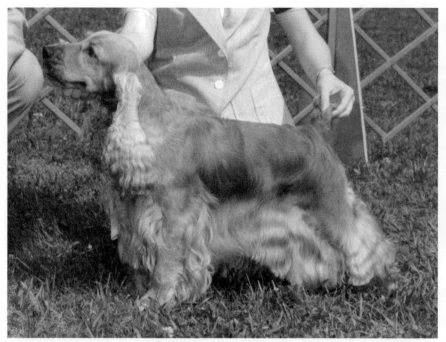

Ch. Gaybrook Amber of Hobbithill, red bitch (Ch. Sorbrook Dandylion ex Ranzfel Sincerely Amber).

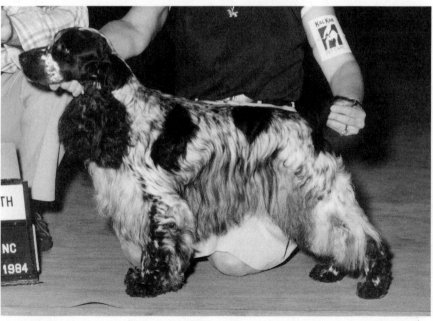

Ch. Chantilly Fire-N-Ice, blue roan dog (Ch. Maidavale Firethorne ex Ch. Dunelm Ladybug).

142

Kermit, a Swedish import who is owned by Mark and Gail, Amber produced nine champions with several more pointed get. From the last breeding of these two Cockers came their most famous son, Am. & Can. Ch. Hobbithill Ashwood Hi Class, the Best of Breed winner at the 1986 American Spaniel Club show and Canada's all-breed top show dog in 1986.

A few words about their other star, Ch. Hubbestad Kermit. In limited stud use Kermit is, to date, the sire of fifteen American and Canadian champions, with six additional pointed offspring.

Hobbithill has produced a total of twelve champions—nine American and three Canadian, with at least nine other offspring pointed.

Joyce Dowling, Florida: Kenmare

Joyce got a quick start in the breed when in 1978 she purchased a young pointed dog named Somerset's Blue Omega from his breeders, Gail Holda and Barbara Gamache. Blue Omega completed his championship very quickly and Joyce was hooked. Another call to Gail Holda to acquire a foundation bitch produced Ch. Somerset's Blue Cricket (Ch. Kenobo Capricorn ex Ch. Somerset Saga's Antigone), who finished from the Puppy class at ten months of age.

Cricket was bred to several notable sires. One of these was Ch. Birchwyn Welshguard. From this breeding came Ch. Kenmare's Lovegift and Ch. Kenmare's Ringbearer. Another breeding, to Ch. Camberle Nightlife, produced Ch. Kenmare's Night Ranger. Both of these litters consisted of only two puppies in each.

One of the most significant litters Cricket had, and one that affected Kenmare in a most positive way, was the breeding to Ch. Winsonem Windstar Major. From this breeding came Ch. Kenmare's Major Motion, Ch. Kenmare's Justa Swingin and Kenmare's What a Feeling.

Not to be outdone by his kennelmate Cricket, Ch. Somerset's Blue Omega has proven his worth as a sire. He has sired, among others, Ch. Lord Charlton of Kenmare, a striking black and white dog; and Kenmare's Blue Scherzo, or "Bess," as she is called.

Since showing was not Bess's idea of fun, she has remained home and has made a very positive contribution to Kenmare as a mother, having produced Ch. Kenmare's Blueberry Nibbles and several other pointed get.

Barbara R. Dzbinski, Maryland: Boxhill

Barbara Dzbinski's Boxhill Kennels is a small, selective breeding and showing hobby kennel located in Maryland. Barbara's first English Cocker, acquired in 1978, was a blue roan bitch, Gunpowder's Maggie Mae. Under Barbara's guidance, "Maggie" quickly attained her American and Canadian CD.

Maggie was bred to a black and white German import, Aro's Pam Pam. From that breeding came an orange and white dog, Ch. Boxhill's Maro's Venture, and a blue roan and tan bitch, Ch. Boxhill's Kodachrome, who became the foundation of the Boxhill line.

As of April 1989 Barbara has bred eight American and Canadian champions, with several other young dogs major pointed. Barbara's greatest thrill was to finish Ch. Boxhill's Bewitched, completely owner handled from the Bred by Exhibitor class. Barbara feels that quality breeding, not quantity breeding, is her most positive contribution to the breed.

Judy and Loyd Eaton, South Carolina: Chantilly

After having Irish Setters for several years, Loyd and Judy started looking for a smaller breed. In 1987 they purchased two English Cocker bitches from Arthur and Jane Ferguson of Dunelm Kennels. With these two bitches, Dunelm Lucinda and Dunelm Ladybug, Loyd and Judy got off to a flying start. Lucinda finished within the year and was bred only once, to Ch. Reklawholm Firebird. This breeding produced Ch. Chantilly Song-n-Dance Man, Ch. Chantilly Luv-n-Honey, Ch. Chantilly Free-N-Easy, and Ch. Dunelm Mountain Laurel.

Ladybug completed her championship with three major wins. Bred to Ch. Maidavale Firethorne she produced Ch. Chantilly Fire-N-Ice, a Group winner and multi-Group placer. Fire-N-Ice sired Chantilly Sport-n-Life, an orange and white dog who finished with four major wins from the Bred by Exhibitor class, a real thrill for any breeder! Fire-N-Ice also sired Ch. Berridale Dream Come True, a blue roan and tan Group-winning dog.

To date, Chantilly has produced eight champions from only four litters. All of these dogs have been owner handled.

Ann Eldredge, Virginia: Maidavale

In 1973 Ann Eldredge was given an English Cocker as an anniversary present from her husband, Ted, a well-known breeder of

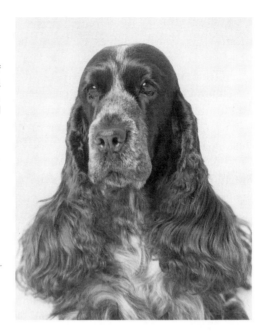

Ch. Springfield's Maggie of Dunde, blue roan bitch (Am. & Can. Ch. Ranzfel Newsflash, Am. & Can. TD, ex Ch. Springfield Brocade, Am. & Can. CD).

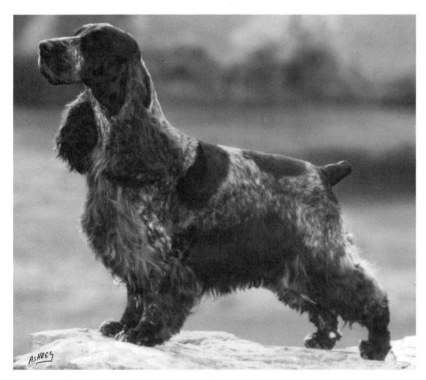

Ch. Maidavale Firefly, blue roan bitch (Ch. Reklawholm Firebird ex Ch. Maidavale Tiffin).
John L. Ashbey

145

Irish Setters under the Tirvelda prefix. Surrey Blue Jean, purchased from Mr. and Mrs. James E. Clark, became the first champion and the foundation bitch for Maidavale Kennels.

Blue was bred twice to Ch. Dunelm Galaxy and from these breedings came eight American champions and one Canadian. Whelped in the first litter was Ch. Maidavale St. Margaret of Ives ("Maggy"), who at the time was only the second English Cocker bitch in the breed's history to win a Best in Show.

Maggy's litter sister, Ch. Maidavale Tiffin, a blue roan and tan bitch, proved to be the next prepotent bitch in the kennel. Her legacy, among others, was Ch. Maidavale Firefly and Ch. Maidavale Firethorne, both sired by Ch. Reklawholm Firebird. Firefly was the top English Cocker bitch in 1979, and Firethorne became a top stud dog a few years later, having sired over thirty champions.

Ann also bought Ch. Sunset's Maidavale Triumph, the tricolored son of Ch. Kenobo Rabbit of Nadou. From Triumph descended two other excellent producers, Ch. Dunelm Nutbrown Maid, co-owned with Jane Ferguson; and Ch. Dunelm Flourish of Tirvelda, owned at one time by Arthur Ferguson and Ted Eldredge.

The black and tan Ch. Kenobo Capricorn son, Ch. Charlton's Maidavale Tanbark, was also purchased, as was the lovely Ch. Reklawholm Lyric of Ranzfel, bred by Prudence Walker and owned at the time by Virginia Lyne. Lyric in turn sired Ch. Maidavale Rosafe Citation, a black and white dog who also figures strongly in the history of Maidavale. Rosie sired many champions, including Ch. Fieldstone Black-Eyed Susan, owned by Connie Vanacore and Mary Ann Alston, and Ch. Fieldstone Bachelor Button, who is owned by Nancy Case.

Ch. Maidavale Night Flight, a blue roan dog sired by Ch. Perrocay Curzon Corregidor out of Ch. Maidavale Fly By Night, is one of the current residents of Maidavale. Night Flight acquired two Group placements from the classes on his march to his championship and has several champion offspring to his credit.

Sue Ernst, Illinois: Aberdeen

In 1979 Sue purchased her foundation bitch from Jane Bond. This bitch, Ch. Springfield's Maggie of Dunde quickly finished her championship at fourteen months of age. From her first litter, sired by Ch. Candleshoes Bayberry Wax, five puppies out of a total of six completed their championships. Among those five are Ch. Aberdeen's Scotch Whiskey, Ch. Aberdeen's Highland Tweed and Ch. Aberdeen's

Royal Sterling. Maggie was a top producing dam in 1983 and 1986, with eight out of a total of seventeen puppies completing their championships.

Maggie's daughter, Ch. Aberdeen's Penyanne of Sequoia, has produced six champions in two litters, with several more only needing a major win to finish. Penyanne is owned by Ellen Vayda.

In 1983, 1986 and 1987 Sue Ernst was one of several top English Cocker breeders of record.

Randall Feather and Martin Sellers, Pennsylvania: Stage Door

Randy and Martin began Stage Door English Cockers in 1979 with the purchase of the puppy who became Ch. Foxfrye's Stage Door Johnny (Ch. Dunelm Guardsman ex Ch. Wingslade on Parade of Foxfyre) from Mary Ann Foxwell. Johnny quickly made his mark by winning Best of Breed at the 1981 National Specialty, and then went on to a successful show career in the United States before being sold to Hedy Hermon of São Paulo, Brazil, where he sired several Brazilian champions.

Ch. Somerset's Stage Door Review (Ch. Kenobo Rabbit of Nadou ex Ch. Somersets-Saga Antigone) was another top winning dog purchased by Randy and Martin. He was whelped in April 1980, achieved notable success in the show ring and is the sire of eleven champions to date.

The foundation bitch at Stage Door is Ch. Log Tavern Stage Door Debut (Ch. Kenobo Capricorn ex Ch. Log Tavern Phara Sunshine), bred by Betty Bathgate and whelped in February 1982. Debut won Best of Breed at the 1983 National Specialty and has produced five champions to date, all of which are bitches; four are Group placers. Her litter by Ch. Olde Spice Crusader, whelped in August 1984, contained four champion bitches: Ch. Stage Door's Summerfield Debut, Ch. Stage Door's Opening Night, Ch. Stage Door's Log Tavern Charade and Ch. Stage Door's Log Tavern Crystal.

Debut's litter by Ch. Lynann's Risky Business, born in November 1987, contained the precocious bitch, Ch. Stage Door's Runaway Bride, who was a Group winner before she was one year old. Randy considers Bride to be his best English Cocker yet. She was Best in Futurity at the English Cocker Spaniel Club of America Futurity in February 1989, and has other Group placements and several breed and Best of Opposite Sex awards, all before the age of two.

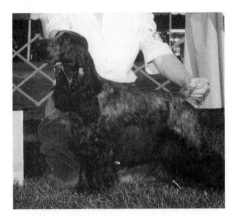

Ch. Stage Door's Runaway Bride, blue roan bitch (Ch. Lynann's Risky Business ex Ch. Log Tavern Stage Door Debut). *Ashbey Photography*

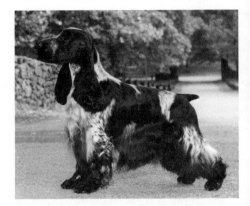

Ch. Somerset's Stage Door Review, blue roan dog (Ch. Kenobo Rabbit of Nadou ex Ch. Somerset's Saga Antigone). *John L. Ashbey*

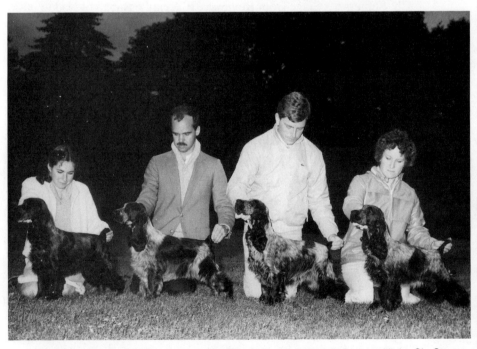

Left to right: Ch. Stage Door's Summerfield Debut, Ch. Stage Door's Opening Night, Ch. Stage Door's Log Tavern Crystal and Ch. Stage Door's Log Tavern Charade.

148

Arthur and Jane Ferguson, North Carolina: Dunelm

Both Arthur and Jane Ferguson enjoyed the companionship of dogs from childhood, but it was not until after World War II that the couple began to raise English Cockers seriously. In 1955 they bought a male puppy, who became Joyanne's Daniel of Dunelm ("Danny"). He was a son of the top winning Ch. Elblac's Bugle of Hastern. The same year they imported a bitch from England, who was in whelp to Colinwood Blazeaway. The bitch, Woodroyd Carousel ("Tess"), became one of the top producers in the breed, with eleven champions, including Ch. Dunelm Pygmalion, who was the sire of Ch. Dunelm Galaxy. Five of Tess's champions were by Blazeaway, the rest by Danny. Most of the Dunelm dogs trace to those two matings.

The Fergusons continued to breed a succession of good dogs, but were concerned that the American dogs were becoming too exaggerated in comparison to the compact, all-of-a-piece, unexaggerated elegance that they felt, and continue to feel, is the proper English Cocker. In 1972 they acquired a dog from Prudence Walker (Reklawholm), who was to play a significant part in their breeding program. He was Ch. Reklawholm Firebird, an orange roan dog who during his career sired more than sixty champions.

Their most interesting litter was by Pygmalion out of Ch. Dunelm Stardust (Ch. Glengaddon Lucky Star ex Dunelm Merry-go-round). This was the litter that contained Galaxy, Galatea and the dark-blue and tan Trick or Treat. This blending of their original stock with the style and temperament of Lucky Star gave them the elegance with the compact bodies they desired.

The Fergusons have continued to combine the same basic lines, with an occasional outcross, resulting in more than 116 champions and still counting. Arthur's advice to prospective breeders is to think three generations back and two ahead. Stay within a line that seems to work, but do not inbreed within the immediate family without very good reason.

The most important thing to look for in a dog is balance, Arthur believes, meaning that the relations of parts to the whole results in a dog that looks right both mechanically and aesthetically, one in which the whole is greater than the sum of its parts. The most objectionable faults, he feels, are poor temperament, long backs, bad topline, receding skulls and common expression.

The Fergusons' primary interest has been in breeding. They are particularly proud of their bitch line, including such excellent producers as Dorinda, Galatea, Indigo Bunting and Starlet. As a rule the Fer-

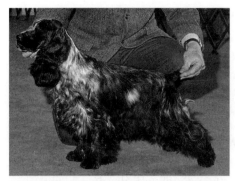

Ch. Dunelm Indigo Bunting, blue roan bitch (Ch. Reklawholm Firebird ex Ch. Dunelm Starlet).
Earl Graham

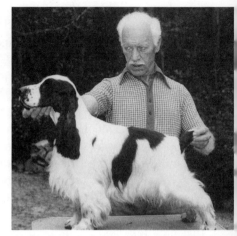

Ch. Dunelm Hallmark, black and white dog (Ch Reklawholm Firebird ex Dunelm Blossom).

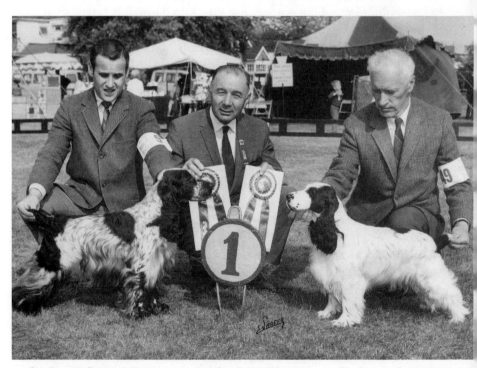

Ch. Dunelm Galaxy *(left)*, blue roan dog (Ch. Dunelm Pygmalion ex Ch. Dunelm Stardust), and Ch. Dunelm Samantha, black and white bitch (Ch. Silver Lariot of Strathpine ex Dunelm Pandora).
Evelyn M. Shafer

150

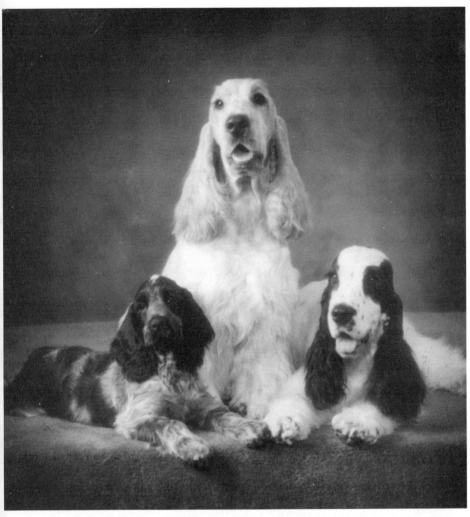

Left to right: Lynann's Sapphire Cinders (Ch. Olde Spice Crusader ex Ch. Lynann's Precious Image), Ch. Songbird's Firefall Embers (Ch. Shaemar Timmara Fyrebrand ex Ch. Winsonem Shadow Dancer) and Ch. Medley Major Motion (Ch. Ranzfel Highlight ex Ch. Winsonem Shadow Dancer).

151

gusons do not keep males, although they are naturally proud of Galaxy's record, succeeded only by his grandson, Capricorn.

Thirty-six of the bitches bred by the Fergusons have produced one or more champions, and of these at least twenty-three have produced three or more; at least thirteen, five or more.

The Fergusons, now in their fourth decade, continue to produce sound, typey English Cockers that will continue to have an important influence on the breed for generations to come.

Jan and Mark Fleming, California: Songbird

While attending the 1979 English Cocker National Specialty, Jan was attracted to the light blue roan dogs of Winsonem Kennels. She picked out Ch. Applewyn Angus (the father of the Winsonem dogs that she admired) as her favorite for Best of Breed and was very excited to see him win that honor. Several months later, she acquired a puppy from Larry and Sandy Sims of Winsonem Kennels. That puppy, Ch. Winsonem Shadow Dancer ("Jessie") became their foundation bitch.

Jessie proved to be an excellent brood bitch. Her five champion offspring include Ch. Songbird's Jumpin Jack Flash, sired by Winsonem Corn Fritter; Ch. Medley Major Motion, co-bred with Marsha Williams; Ch. Medley Emily Regan of Massac, also co-bred with Marsha; Ch. Songbird's Firefall Embers; and Ch. Medley's Megaton of Ritchaven, a son of Ch. Paganhill Persuasion.

Jan's hobby is drawing, and her drawings of English Cockers can be seen in many places, including on stationery and on a cover for the *English Cocker Quarterly* magazine.

Mary Ann Foxwell, Maryland: Foxfyre

The Foxfyre English Cockers were shown simultaneously with Foxfyre Irish Setters for several years. Mary Ann's first English Cocker, Ch. Kenobo Foxfyre Fascination, was purchased in 1973, followed by her foundation bitch, Ch. Wingslade On Parade of Foxfyre, bred by Sandra Sisson. An excellent producer, she gave Foxfyre its first homebred English Cocker champion, Foxfyre Spellbound O'Tomeran, owned by Phyllis Floyd. In her second litter, sired by Ch. Dunelm Guardsman, she produced the 1981 National Specialty winner, Ch. Foxfyre Stagedoor Johnny, a top breed winner. At that time Johnny was owned by Randall Feather and Martin Sellers.

Ch. Dragonhold's F'lessa O'Foxfyre, a litter sister to Stagedoor

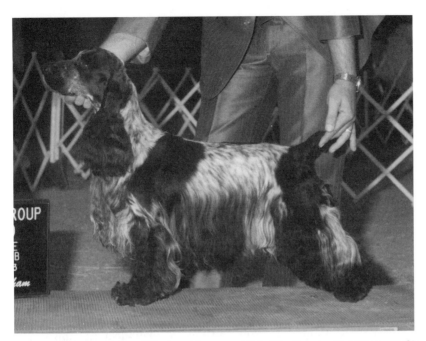

Ch. Dragonhold's Flessa O'Foxfyre, blue roan bitch (Ch. Dunelm Guardman ex Ch. Wingslade On Parade of Foxfyre).

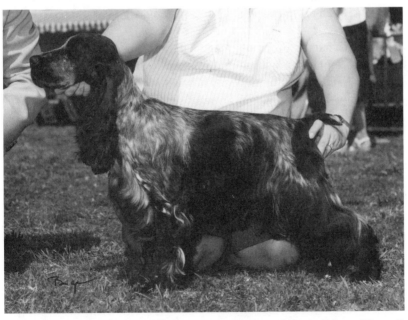

Ch. Lynann's Precious Image, blue roan bitch (Ch. Glenwood's Sierra Echo ex Wyncastle Cinderella). *Rich Bergman Photos*

Johnny, also did her share of winning with Bests of Breed and Group placements to her credit. She is a top producer, with three current champions to her credit, all Group placers.

Foxfyre's Shady Lady, bred twice to Ch. Trupence Fife and Drum, produced several orange roan champions, including Ch. Foxfyre's Funny Valentine, owned by Sally Gray, and Ch. Foxfyre's Fieldstone Phoenix, an orange roan male co-owned by Dale Hood and Mary Ann Alston, who completed his championship with a Group placement.

In recent years, Mary Ann has added solid colors to her kennel and has produced the black dog Ch. Foxfyre All Flags Flying.

Foxfyre Kennels strives to breed elegant, balanced English Cockers with good movement and temperament. This is reflected in the twenty-three champions that Foxfyre has produced and Mary Ann twice being named the top breeder of English Cockers in the United States.

Lynda and Robert Gall, California: Lynann

The first English Cocker and the foundation of Lynann was a small dark-blue roan bitch by the name of Wyncastle Cinderella. Bred to Ch. Glenwood's Sierra Echo, Cinders produced Ch. Lynann's Quicksilver and Ch. Lynann's Repeat Performance, and the multiple Best of Breed–winning and Group-placing Ch. Lynann's Precious Image.

Ch. Lynann's Precious Image easily finished her championship, at thirteen months of age, at the Southern California Specialty show. Bred to Ch. Old Spice Crusader, this beautiful blue roan bitch produced four champion offspring: Ch. Lynann's Never Ending Story; Ch. Lynann's Risky Business; Ch. Lynann's Pacific Pizzazz; and Ch. Lynann's Sapphire Cinders, who was Best of Winners at the English Cocker National Specialty in St. Louis.

Betty Ganung, New York: Amawalk

Rusty, a deep-orange and white male, came to Amawalk at eight weeks of age, and though never bred, he was the beginning of Betty's love of English Cockers.

In 1974 Betty set off on a hunt for the perfect foundation bitch for her Amawalk Kennels. Betty acquired Ancram Muffin of Amawalk, who produced one litter. From that litter of five, sired by Ch. Kenobo Constellation, a bitch puppy was kept. This puppy, who became Ch. Amawalk Lucky Charm, was the true foundation stone for Amawalk.

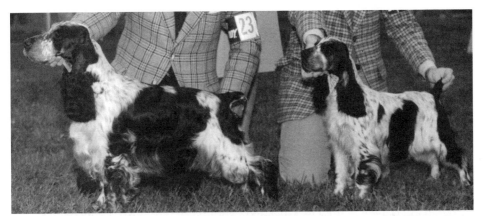

Ch. Amawalk's Cottleston Concorde *(left)*, blue roan and tan dog, with littermate Ch. Amawalk's Flying Colors, blue roan and tan bitch (Ch. Dunelm Galaxy ex Ch. Amawalk's Lucky Charm).

William P. Gilbert

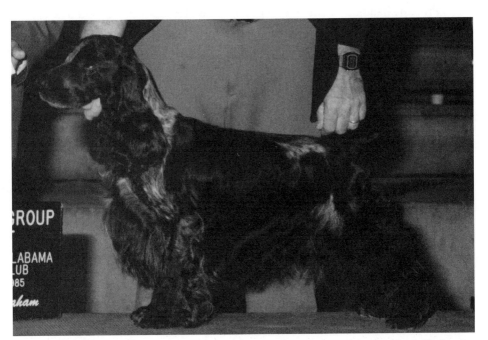

Ch. Gala Glen Vatican Soldier, blue roan dog (Ch. Gala Glen Bluejay ex Ch. Meadowlark's Stacy O'Gala Glen).

Earl Graham Studios

155

From her first litter, sired by Ch. Dunelm Galaxy, came two champions, both of whom were blue roan and tan. The first, Ch. Amawalk Cottleston Concorde, became Betty's first champion, finishing at eleven months of age. After a very respectable show career he was sent to Venezuela, where he became a top-ranked Sporting dog. He returned to the States and sired several notable dogs, including Ch. Bluebell Irish Tweed and Ch. Bluebell Dark Crystal. His sister, Ch. Amawalk Flying Colors, in turn produced three champions for Amawalk.

Lucky Charm produced a total of five champions. Her daughter, from her last litter by Ch. Springfield Michelob, won the Winners Bitch class at the first Canadian English Cocker Specialty show. This liver roan bitch, Ch. Amawalk's Darkenwald Bettina, CD, TD, WD, is owned by Carol Richter of Washington State.

One of Betty's favorites, Ch. Amawalk's Katrina, another Lucky Charm daughter sired by Ch. Reklawholm Firebird, also produced five champions. Katrina's son by Ch. Kenobo Confetti, Ch. Perrocay Qeqertaq ("Pacman"), has the enviable record of being the number one owner-handled dog for three years straight. During this time, his owner, Scott Proctor, handled Pacman to over a hundred Group placings and a Best in Show. Pacman's litter brother, Ch. Amawalk's Questrist, also placed in the top rankings for English Cockers for the year 1984 in just several months of showing.

Katrina's last litter, sired by Ch. Edgewood Fan Tan, produced Ch. Amawalk's Xtravaganza and Ch. Amawalk's Xecutive Miss, both of whom completed their championships at very young ages with impressive wins.

To date Amawalk has bred or co-bred twenty-two champions. Many of the Amawalk dogs carry obedience and field degrees, an accomplishment of which Betty is very proud.

John and Carolanne Garlick and Constance Boldt, Florida: Sher-Ron

The story of John and Carolanne's involvement with the breed begins in 1981, when they acquired Gala Glen Vatican Soldier. Soldier easily completed his championship in seven shows, and although shown only sparingly, this multi-Group winner became a top-ranked English Cocker for three consecutive years. He has proven to be a prepotent sire, with fifteen champions and many other pointed children to his credit.

Jean Glassen, Michigan: Maple Lawn

The first English Cocker to join the family of Jean and Hal Glassen and their household of English Setters was Basquaerie Blue of Robwood. Although this bitch was not a good producer, she became the entree for the Glassens to become involved in English Cocker activities. This was during World War II.

In 1958 they imported the dog that became the foundation for Maple Lawn, Ch. Lochnell Blue Flash of Ulwell, a blue roan dog. During the following years, four bitches were imported to breed to this dog, and all Maple Lawn English Cockers descend from these original imports, all of whom came from the Lochnell Kennels. Among the most notable is Ch. Maple Lawn Slumber Party, a black and white bitch by Ch. Maple Lawn Jaunti Jactation out of Ch. Maple Lawn Day Dreamer, whelped in 1966. She was the dam of fourteen champions. Several other Maple Lawn bitches produced multiple champions, among them Day Dreamer and Silk and Silver. Maple Lawn continues today with offspring of Ch. Maple Lawn Parade Strutter, who has been bred to Ch. Olde Spice Crusader and more recently to Ch. Maple Lawn Jim Brady's Gem.

More than fifty champions carry the Maple Lawn prefix, although the Glassens raise only two or three litters per year.

Phyllis Goldberg, Oregon: Tin Star

Phyllis has been showing Sporting dogs since moving to Oregon from Chicago in 1972. At that time she handled Irish Setters in breed competition, obedience and field. In 1976 she added English Cockers to her household and has been quite successful with her breeding program thus far. In 1986 she was runner-up for breeder of the year, as well as owning a top-ranked brood bitch, Ch. Tin-Star's My Lil' Chickadee.

Chickadee is the dam of the following champions to date: Ch. Tin-Star's Classy Chassis, sired by Camberle Fiddler on the Ruff; and sired by Ch. Kenobo Capricorn are Ch. Tin-Star's Captain Marvel (co-owned with Margaret Hadaway), Ch. Tin-Star's Diamond of Paganhill (owned by Beth McKinney), Ch. Tin-Star's Knight Rider, CD (owned by Jennifer Degarmo) and Ch. Tin-Star's Front Page, CD (owned by M. Hadaway).

Other noteworthy Tin Star English Cockers include Ch. Tin-Star Mr. T, a dark-blue roan dog; and Cloverleaf N' Tin-Star's Dancer, an orange roan bitch.

Tin Star currently has produced seven champions and four obedience titleholders out of four litters, with several more close to their titles.

Cynthia and Haywood Harrell, Arizona: Delashire

Under the tutelage of dog trainer Max Parris, Cynthia Harrell took her first English Cocker, Delashire Journey South, all the way to the coveted Obedience Trial Championship title. Her subsequent accomplishments with two other all-breed High in Trial winners marked her as one of the premier English Cocker obedience handlers of the 1980s. Over a five-year period between 1981 and 1986, out of twelve English Cocker Specialties entered, Cynthia and Woody Harrell's dogs accumulated nine High in Trials and two Highest Scoring wins.

Delashire Journey South was the offspring of an English mother from the Patbarossa Kennel and has close ties to Mrs. duPont's Squirrel Run Kennel. One of Journey's strengths was his competitiveness in obedience runoffs. His finest effort in this area was a 1982 first-place Open class win from a four-way runoff. However, Journey's 197 score that day proved to be the second highest score by any of the 189 dogs entered and was matched in Novice by his kennelmate Wingslade Southern Colony, who was handled by Woody. The Highest-Scoring dog in the trial that day went to yet another Harrell English Cocker, Wingslade Southern Cause ("Rebel"), who gave Cynthia her first all-breed obedience win with a score of 198 in the Novice B class. This show goes down as one of the breed's finest obedience performances and culminated a season of friendly sibling rivalry between the two Harrell English Cocker entries, both bred by Sandra Sisson.

The blue roan and tan Rebel became the breed's youngest obedience Specialty winner by taking High in Trial in his first show. Rebel would win the National Specialty twice more, from the Open A class at the 1984 Denver show and from the Open B class in 1986 at the National Specialty fiftieth-anniversary show.

The Harrells called four states home in the 1980s, in conjunction with Woody's career moves with the National Park Services. However they were able to manage two litters by Colony. The first, sired by Ch. Edgewood Play with Fire, CD, TD, produced the dark-blue roan Sojourn Dancing in the Dark. This dog, known as "the Boss," became their fourth dog to win Highest-Scoring Dog in Trial, with a score of 198½ from the Novice B class!

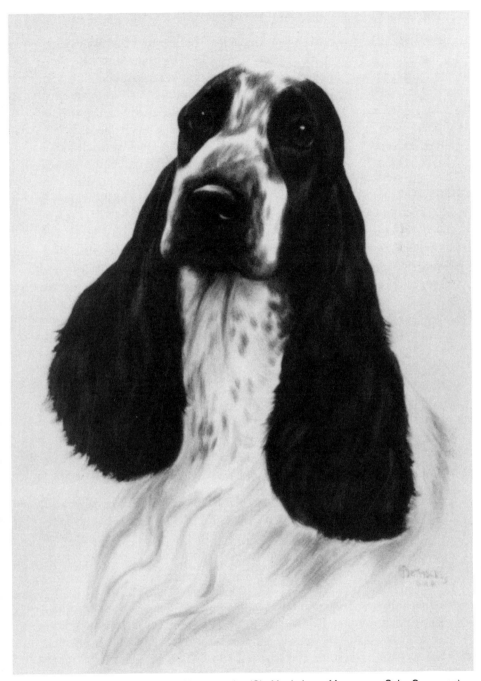

Ch. Soho Marksman of Wyncrest, blue roan dog (Ch. Maple Lawn Magnum ex Soho Sequence).

Barbara Heckerman, Ohio: Wyncrest

Barbara was sixteen years old when she acquired Ch. Soho Nightingale on a co-ownership from Lynn Clark of Soho Kennels. Since Nightingale did not enjoy motherhood, Barbara acquired Soho Sequence for a litter of puppies. From this breeding to Ch. Maple Lawn Magnum came two champions, Wyncrest Ricochet Soho and Soho Marksman of Wyncrest. Marksman had some success in the show ring and more as a remarkable producer whose influence is still felt today.

One of Barbara's favorites, Ch. Wyncrest Windjammer, was a black and white ticked son of Marksman's top producing son, Ch. Soho Counterpoint and Soho Bonus Baby. A breeding of Windjammer to Ch. Soho Spice produced Ch. Wyncrest Windchimes.

Another litter, co-bred with Darlene Andrews and sired by Ch. Wittersham's Emblem and an orange roan Marksman daughter, Mayfair's Marked Card, produced the multiple Best in Show Ch. Mayfair-Wyncrest Baccarat and Ch. Mayfair-Wyncrest Roulette. A lovely red male, Wyncrest-Mayfair Talisman, is the result of a breeding of Roulette to Am. & Can. Ch. Bryansbrook High Society.

On both a professional and personal level, Barbara's close association with, among others, Soho and Wittersham Kennels, has given her the expertise and opportunity to guide the show careers of some truly great dogs. Even though Barbara has not bred many litters, she is pleased that Wyncrest has produced four quality generations of English Cockers.

Maureen Helbig, New York: Arigna

The Arigna Kennel of Maureen Helbig originated in 1974 with the acquisition of Coconia Bye Bye Blues from Anne Labouchere. This black and white ticked bitch lived fifteen years and was the great-grandmother of the 1987 National Sweepstakes winner Ch. Arigna Avatar Tartan, a Ch. Edgewood Fan Tan daughter.

In 1983 Maureen had the good fortune of purchasing a five-month-old orange roan bitch from the Gunpowder Kennels of Barbara Tucci MacDougall. This bitch, Gunpowder's Arigna Pippin completed her championship very easily and was bred to Ch. Cedarhurst Jonathan Seagull. From this match came the 1985 National Specialty Winners Dog, Ch. Gunpowder's Arigna Golion.

Ch. Edgewood Fan Tan came to live with Maureen in the fall of 1984. Bred by Mark and Bonnie Threlfall, he completed his cham-

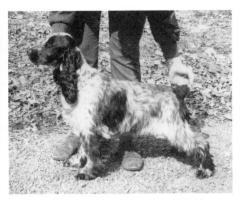

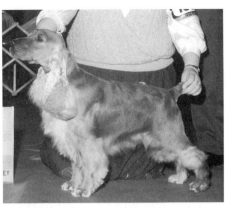

Am. & Can. Ch. Mayfair Wyncrest Baccarat, red dog (Ch. Wittersham's Emblem ex Mayfair Marked Card). *Ashbey Photography*

Ch. Dunelm Starlet, blue roan bitch (Ch. Dunelm Galaxy ex Ch. Dunelm Dorinda).

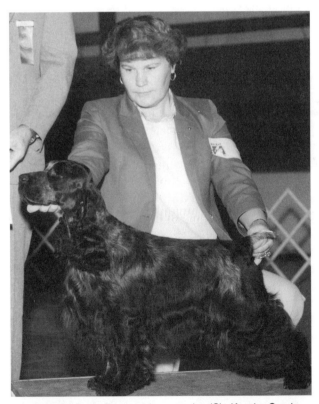

Ch. Malagold Storm Trooper, blue roan dog (Ch. Kenobo Capricorn ex Ch. Malagold's Molly). *Cott/Daigle*

161

pionship with three five-point major wins. He went on to win Best of Opposite Sex at the National Specialty in 1985 and again in 1986. In 1987 and 1988 he topped them all by winning Best of Breed at the National Specialty, thus being the first dog in the history of the breed to be the top male at a National Specialty for four consecutive years. In 1987 he was a top producer, with seven champions to his credit.

Carole Hoke, Washington: Linarca

Carole Hoke and Lincara began in 1970 with the purchase of Crickora Fancy Feathers. Fancy Feathers completed her championship and attained a CD in obedience. She was bred four times and produced two champions and several more pointed get. While stationed in England with her husband, who was in the air force, Carole showed Ch. Linarcas Sodalite and won several Bests of Breed over the English dogs. Back in the United States again, this international dog capped his career with a BOB and Group IV from the Veteran class. He was ten years old at the time.

Dr. James Holt, Virginia: Meadowfarm

Jim acquired his first English Cocker in 1970 from Arthur and Jane Ferguson. She was Ch. Dunelm Georgie Girl, a black and white bitch who was about four years old at the time and in whelp to Ch. Reklawholm Paul Jones. Her sweet personality inserted a "hook" into Jim that still holds to this day.

"Georgie" had six male puppies from that breeding. One puppy, Ch. Meadowfarm's Cinders on Snow, Jim kept and finished. Another puppy, Ch. Meadowfarm's Most Happy Fella, was sold to Roberta and Bob Benvin of Of Sorts Kennel. The two brothers were occasionally shown as a brace, and being nearly mirror image black and white, made a very striking pair that won several all-breed Best Brace in Show awards, as well as Best Brace at an English Cocker National Specialty.

Jim's next acquisition was Ch. Dunelm Starlet ("Lettie"), from Arthur and Jane Ferguson. Lettie was bred to Ch. Reklawholm Firebird, and out of that litter came Ch. Dunelm Meadowfarm Flicker and Ch. Dunelm Indigo Bunting. After her puppies were dispersed, Lettie returned to the Fergusons. However, she put on such a performance of English "high pout," refusing to eat and sitting with her back to the other dogs and her nose in a corner of the yard, that very soon

Jim got a call from Arthur and Jane asking him if Lettie could "come home."

Lettie came home and was bred again to Ch. Reklawholm Firebird, and from that litter came Ch. Meadowfarm Bluejay, a dog that Jim kept. Lettie is on the list of top producers in the breed and at least for a while was Ch. Dunelm Galaxy's top producing daughter.

Next came a blue roan and tan bitch as a birthday present to Jim. She became Ch. Meadowfarm Wedgewood Robin and in turn produced Meadowfarm Rosie the Riveter, CDX, TDX, sired by Ch. Maidavale Rosafe Citation.

Jim serves as the English Cocker Spaniel Club of America's AKC Delegate and is a member of the Board of Directors of the American Kennel Club.

Mary Hopkins, Wisconsin: Morningside

Mary received her first English Cocker as a birthday gift in 1976. This birthday gift, a four-month-old puppy bred by Mary Ann Alston, grew up to be Ch. Fieldstone Blu Sky, CD. "Sky" acquired several Group placements in a short career and achieved his CD obedience degree in three shows.

In 1982 Mary bred Ch. Malagold's Molly, CD, who was co-owned with Dirk Benson, to Ch. Kenobo Capricorn. From this breeding came Ch. Malagold's Storm Trooper, a Group winner and multiple-champion-producing stud.

Pat Janzen, Colorado

Pat's involvement with solid English Cockers began in 1981 when she acquired Ch. Fireside Yes I Can, WD, a black dog. He won the 1982 National Futurity and finished before he turned a year old. He earned his WD and went on to earn multiple Group placements.

In 1982, Pat acquired Ch. Hobbithill Ebonwood's Ember, a red bitch. She produced two champions (both red dogs) from her first litter by Ch. Lorjo's Something Smashing, Ch. Ebonwood Crackerjack and Ch. Ebonwood's Chief Contender, CD. Pat has also imported two red bitches from well-known English kennels. Ch. Kavora Copyright finished in only two months, and her first litter produced three champions and several obedience-titled English Cockers. The other import, Am. & Can. Ch. Lochdene Mini Cheddar, finished with two BOBs and a Group II placement.

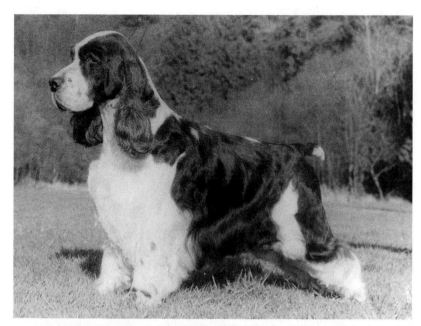

Am. & Can. Ch. Wingslade Kvammes Spirit, WDX, TD, black and white male (Ch. Kenobo Capricorn ex Ch. Kenobo Touch of Majic).

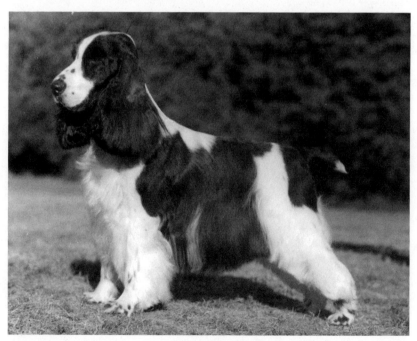

Am. & Can. Ch. Kvammes Razzle Dazzle, WDX, TD, black and white bitch (Am. & Can. Ch. Wingslade Kvammes Spirit, WDX, TD, ex Ch. Kvamme's Astral, TD).

164

Linda Klaers, Minnesota: Linmark

Obedience showing is where Linda Klaers is most interested, and in this area she has enjoyed much success. One reason for this success is OTCH. Old Spice Royal Commander, UD. The journey to his Utility Dog degree is quite impressive. Along the way he garnered four first place finishes in Novice, ten first place finishes in Open, and nine first place finishes in Utility. He went High in Trial on three separate occasions before he acquired his UD. He completed the requirements for his Obedience Trial Championship (OTCH) in May of 1987.

Also residing at Linmark is Olde Spice Stormy Sea, who has begun her quest for a breed championship with a major win and will compete in both obedience and field competition in the future.

Lorrie and Marlin Kvamme, Washington: Kvamme

Marlin and Lorrie's story begins where so many other stories begin, with another breed, usually a Sporting dog and usually a big dog. In Marlin's case it began with Golden Retrievers and much success with that breed. However, Marlin and Lorrie wanted a smaller house dog and were drawn to the English Cocker because they are very much a big dog in a small-dog package. The Kvammes give credit to such top kennels as Dunelm, Kenobo, Maidavale, Reklawholm, and Wingslade for their success today.

Am. & Can. Ch. Wingslade Kvammes Spirit, WDX, TD, bred by and co-owned with Sandra Sisson, although disliking the show ring, completed both his American and Canadian championships easily. However, Spirit's real passion was field work and this he proved by being the first English Cocker in the West to complete his WDX. Although he was only used on a limited stud basis, he is the sire of numerous Specialty winners.

Am. & Can. Ch. Kvamme's Astral, TD, was Marlin and Lorrie's first homebred. Astral was owner handled to number three bitch in the country during 1981, even though taking time out for maternal duties. Astral made history by winning Best of Opposite Sex at the British Columbia Cocker Specialty for three consecutive years. Astral's sire was Am. & Can. Ch. Copperally Minstral of Reklawholm, and her dam was Can. Ch. Wingslade Blue Silk N' Saffron. Astral was a prepotent producer and is the dam of Am. & Can. Ch. Kvammes Razzle Dazzle, WDX, TD; Am. & Can. Ch. Kvammes Star Dust, WDX, TD; and Ch. Kvammes Sun Dance, among others.

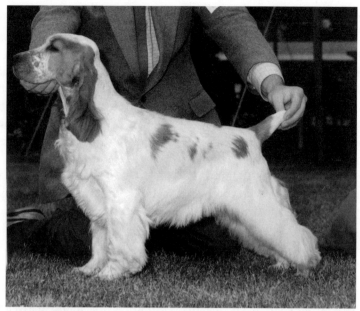

Ch. Kvammes High Style, orange roan bitch (Ch. Olde Spice Crusader ex Am. & Can. Ch. Kvammes Razzle Dazzle, WDX, TD). *Charles Tatham*

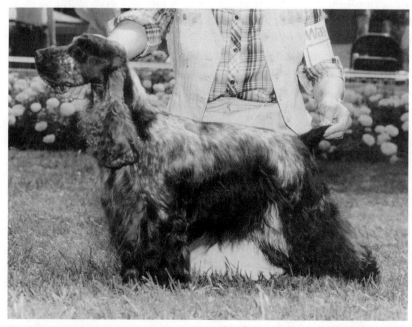

Ch. Carra-Lee Midnight Lace, blue roan bitch (Ch. Graecroft Tarus of Wyncastle ex Ch. Carra-Lee Auntie Mame). *MikRon Photos*

166

Although Marlin and Lorrie have bred many beautiful Cockers and have had many exciting wins, Ch. Kvammes High Style certainly has provided her share of thrills. Style began her show career by going Best of Winners for a major and on to Best of Breed under noted judge Jane Forsyth. Style's next show was the 1986 National Specialty in Connecticut. There she won the Sweepstakes, went Winners Bitch and Best of Winners and also went Best Puppy! Next came the Santa Barbara Kennel Club show where Style won the breed from the Bred by Exhibitor class over forty-five English Cockers. She finished with her fourth major and fourth Best of Breed from the classes. Style's sire is Am. & Can. Ch. Olde Spice Crusader, and her dam is Am. & Can. Ch. Kvammes Razzle Dazzle, WDX, TD.

Other important Cockers produced by Marlin and Lorrie include Am. & Can. Ch. Kvammes Hollywood, TD, a Specialty winning and champion-producing blue roan dog; Ch. Kvammes Huntress, also a blue roan co-owned with Colleen McKinney, who finished at one year of age; and Ch. Kvammes Keepsake, co-owned with Mary Ann Alston, who finished her championship by going Best of Winners at the 1987 National Specialty.

Carol Lewis, California: Carra-Lee

Carol Lewis and her husband, Robin, began their love affair with dogs in 1962 with the purchase of an Irish Setter. Carol decided to pursue a career as a professional handler and in 1970 was licensed by the AKC. She has been handling professionally ever since.

Her first English Cocker was acquired on a co-ownership from another Irish Setter breeder, Lucy Jane Myers, in 1972. She was an orange roan bitch, Soho Hot Copy ("Mame"), who was more at home in the whelping box than in the show ring. Mame whelped a litter in 1973 that would produce, among others, Ch. Carra-Lee Auntie Mame, a blue roan who in 1978 produced an all-champion litter when bred to Ch. Graecroft Tarus of Wyncastle, a blue roan and tan dog. That litter contained a blue roan bitch, Am. & Mex. Ch. Carra-Lee Midnight Lace; an orange roan bitch, Ch. Carra-Lee Tangerine; and an orange roan dog, Am. & Mex. Ch. Carra-Lee Talk of the Town. Ch. Carra-Lee Tangerine, who was co-owned with Pam Dahl of Timmara Kennel, was bred to Ch. Carachelle Capt. Fantastic and produced Ch. Timmara's New Kid in Town and Ch. Timmara Doolin' Dalton.

Ch. Carra-Lee Midnight Lace was bred to Ch. Glenwood's Indigo Star, a blue roan, to produce the blue roan bitch Ch. Carra-Lee Mood

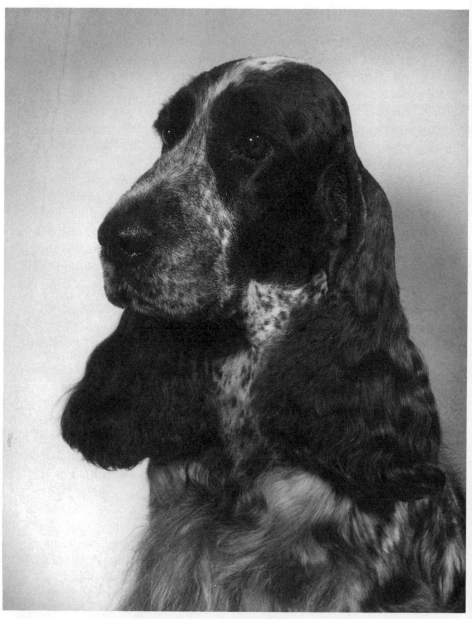

Am. & Can. Ch. Ranzfel Blue Roxanne, blue roan bitch (Ch. Craigleith Magic Flute ex Ranzfel Megan Blue). *Jeradine Lamb*

Indigo. Her final litter, bred to Chitasca Sir Boz O'Wyncastle, produced the pointed "Silver" litter.

A recent breeding at Carra-Lee was a hybrid combination of a liver roan bitch, Ch. Carra-Lee Creme de Cocoa to the red dog Ch. Sorbrook Dandylion. A black bitch from that litter, Carra-Lee Dark Enchantment, is major pointed.

Carol was attracted to the Cockers originally for their merry personalities and their Sporting dog qualities. It is her goal to maintain the "cockery" Cocker, a "true Sporting dog who can do his job if called upon; to maintain the soundness, integrity and type that makes this breed distinctive; and to cherish and preserve the merry temperament of the breed."

Leslie Lockard, Pennsylvania: Brookside

Hunting and field activities are the main focus for Leslie and her Brookside English Cockers. She purchased her first dog in 1980 from the Braeside Kennels of Debbie Mason. She was Braeside Sunlit Brooks, WDX. Brooks's son, Brookside Night Sentinel, is also a WDX and is on his way to being one of the breed's first Junior Hunters.

Leslie belongs to several dog clubs and uses her dogs for field demonstrations and therapy visits.

Virginia Lyne, British Columbia, Canada: Ranzfel

Virginia Lyne has been involved with English Cocker Spaniels as long as she can remember because they were the family pet of choice while she was growing up. Her own first English Cocker, however, did not appear until 1960, when she imported a black-and-white bitch from England. That bitch was Ch. Lochranza Ring Dove. Subsequently Virginia imported a series of English Cockers from England, including the Group-winning Am. & Can. Ch. Colinwood Coastguard, Can. Ch. Colinwood Texan Maid and Can. Ch. Westering Home of Weirdene. Later Virginia added solid-colored English Cockers to Ranzfel with Can. Ch. Lochranza Dancing Mistress and Am. & Can. Ch. Sorbrook Dandylion, a magnificent red dog who enjoyed an illustrious show career both in Canada and the United States.

Ranzfel has produced many notable English Cockers. Among them are Ch. Ranzfel Blue Roxanne, the dam of many champions, including Ch. Ranzfel Newsflash, Am. & Can. TD. Newsflash became the top winning English Cocker in Canada for three years and consistently ranked among the ten top Sporting dogs in Canada. Although shown only sparingly in the United States, he became a multiple breed and Group winner. Aging has been kind to Flash, as he achieved one of his most thrilling wins by going Best of Breed from the Veteran class at the 1984 English Cocker Spaniel Club of America Specialty. He won the Veteran class again at the 1986 National Specialty and delighted the crowd with his enthusiastic performance. In addition to his illustrious show career, Flash acquired both an American and Canadian tracking degree. Flash has also achieved considerable success as a sire, with many Canadian and American champion offspring to his credit.

One of Flash's sons, Ch. Ranzfel Highlight, has several American Bests in Show to his credit. Although not shown often in the States, he did accumulate multiple Group placements, including eight Group firsts. In Canada, where he resides, he has amassed nine all-breed Bests in Show. Highlight has sired several American champions.

One of the latest additions to Ranzfel is Can. & Aus. Ch. Marsden Time Piece, a blue roan dog imported from Phillip Warburton and John Edwards, in Australia.

Over the years Ranzfel has strived to produce a definite type of English Cocker that is distinctive and recognizable as coming from Ranzfel, with temperament being of the utmost importance.

Myra Main, Ontario, Canada: Ashwood

In 1980 Myra and Jim Main bought their first English Cocker, a red puppy, for their daughter, who had complained that the family's German Shepherd Dogs were too big for her to handle.

A year later they purchased Am. & Can. Ch. Wittersham's Excelssimo from Eugene Phoa. This Best in Show dog was bred to their red bitch to produce their first champion, Ashwood's Special Edition, CDX.

Myra's association with the Wittersham kennel continued with the purchase of Am. & Can. Ch. Wittersham Ashwood Captivator, a multiple Best in Show black dog. She purchased a blue roan bitch to breed to Captivator, and that pair produced Am. & Can. Ch. Ashwood Wyncrest Bedazzled, a black bitch who has done quite a bit of winning in the United States and Canada.

In 1984 the puppy whom Myra considers her once-in-a-lifetime dog arrived from the Hobbithill kennel of Mark and Gail Dehayes. He became Am., Can. & Bda. Ch. Hobbithill Ashwood Hi Class, a red

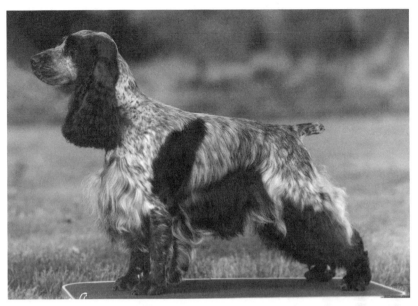

Am. & Can. Ch. Ranzfel Highlight, blue roan dog (Am. & Can. Ch. Ranzfel Newsflash, Am. & Can. TD, ex Ch. Ranzfel Zanzee Blue).   *Animal World Studio © 1985*

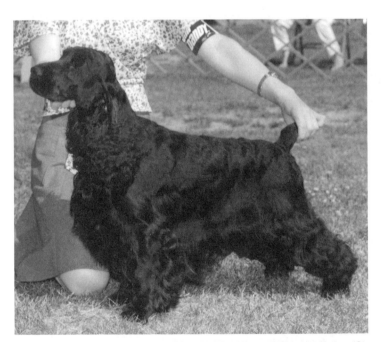

Am., Can. & Bda. Ch. Braeside Dark O' The Moon, WDX, black dog (Ch. Merryborne Minstrel, WDX, Can. WS, ex Shikarwyn's Shooting Star).
William P. Gilbert, Inc.

171

dog of excellent type, conformation and temperament. Hi Class, called Trooper, finished his championship at seven months amassing eighteen Puppy Group Firsts along the way. In 1986, completely owner handled by Mrya, Trooper became the top show dog in Canada, Best of Breed at the American Spaniel Club in New Jersey and an Award of Merit winner at the National Specialty that year. He is now retired, but through selective breeding he has produced several top winning and top producing offspring.

Myra has been also closely associated with the Lochranza kennels in England. She imported a black bitch, Ch. Helmbracken Callie of Lochranza. When bred to Trooper, Callie produced Ch. Ashwood Rather Posh, a black bitch. Myra also imported a famous English show champion, the red dog Lochranza Like Your Style, whom she has incorporated into her line. In 1986 she brought over another red dog, Ch. Lochranza Touching Wood, whom she co-owns with JoAnn Davis and Susan Fiore. Touching Wood had a successful show career in the United States in 1987 and 1988.

Deborah Mason, Massachusetts: Braeside

Debbie Mason has been breeding English Cockers for the better part of twenty years. Her first English Cocker was the black, white and tan Galaxy granddaughter, Fox Rock Carrie of Pinewood. She was the foundation of the Braeside particolor cockers. Her granddaughter, Ch. Braeside Bluebell, has produced seven champions in two litters, sired by Ann Perry's Ch. Ballyweel's Blue Chip, WDX.

Debbie's first solids were the two black dogs, Am. & Can. Ch. Merryborne Minstrel, WDX, Can. WS, and Am. & Can. Ch. Merryborne Miniut, WDX, both bred by Irene Martin, who had just moved from England to the United States. Minstrel earned the distinction of being the first American English Cocker to earn a Working Dog Excellent degree (WDX), a feat he repeated in Canada a week later! Minstrel sired multiple champions, and many of his children have earned field degrees.

One of the most famous Minstrel children was Am., Can. & Bda. Ch. Braeside Dark O' The Moon, WDX. "Sam," as he was best known, was a top ten–ranked English Cocker for five consecutive years, owner handled, and was a multiple Group and Specialty winner. More recent Minstrel children who are proving their worth in the show ring, in the field, and as stud dogs are Ch. Braeside Moongazer, WDX, and Ch. Echilon Braeside Moonraker, WDX, who went Best in Sweepstakes at the 1980 National Specialty.

Striving to maintain type, soundness and temperament, Debbie has imported several dogs from England to blend with her original Merryborne lines. She has imported the black dog Ch. Lochranza Night Patrol, sire of Sunglint, and more recently Ch. Kavora Benito and Kavora Bright Moonlight Bess, respectively a black dog and red bitch by Pam Trotman in England.

Debbie's first red English Cocker, which she co-owned with her mother, Jean, was English import Ch. Merryborne Camille. She is behind almost all of Braeside's current solids. Her grandson, Ch. Merryborne Morning Sunglint, in turn produced Ch. Braeside Belle Mount Spirit, whom Debbie considers one of the best reds she has ever bred. He is a Specialty winner and multiple Group-placing dog and was co-bred with the Burhans.

Barbara McDougall, New Jersey: Gunpowder

Barbara Tucci McDougall has been involved in the breed since 1975, when she acquired her first English Cocker, Ch. Kadon's Touch of Magic, CD, from Kay Monaghan. "Lily," as she was called, became the foundation of Gunpowder Kennels. Lily was bred to Ch. Kenobo Capricorn and presented Barbara with her first homebred, Ch. Gunpowder's Kadon Dee-Dee Dinah, CD, WDX.

Barbara realized her dream of breeding a triple-titled English Cocker with Dinah, and of establishing a line of English Cockers known for their temperament and style. At this same time Barbara experienced a low with the loss of her Best of Breed stud dog, Ch. Gunpowder's Exuberant Godson, who before his death at a young age produced some exceptional pups, who went on to Group wins and championships.

Gunpowder's second litter, by Lily and Ch. Dunelm J. Fred Muggs, produced the lovely orange roan bitch Ch. Gunpowder's Kadon Susie Q., CD. A third litter, by Lily and Ch. Reklawholm Firebird, yielded a striking light-blue roan dog who finished easily, Ch. Gunpowder's Flint and Steel.

Gunpowder has produced many other champions, including Ch. Gunpowder's Encore of Sunspan, Ch. Gunpowder's Han'som Headliner and Ch. Gunpowder Arigna Pippin.

Beth C. McKinney, Washington: Paganhill

The Paganhill Kennel of Beth McKinney traces its beginning to 1966, when Beth purchased Soho Speculation from Lynn Clark. Beth

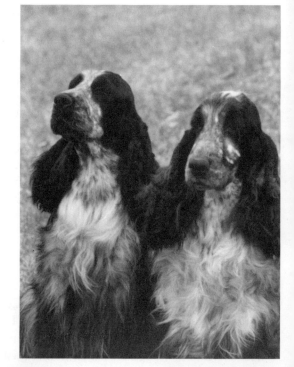

Ch. Gunpowder's Kadon Dee-D-Dinah, CD, WDX *(left)*, and Ch. Kadon's Touch of Magic, CD.

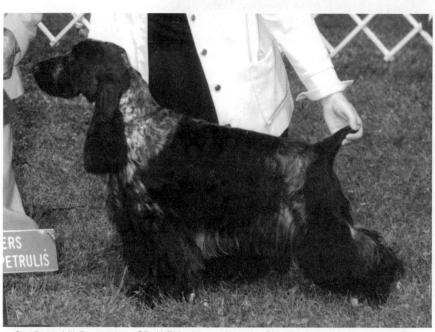

Ch. Paganhill Persuasion, CD, WDX, blue roan bitch (Ch. Maidavale Firethorne ex Ch. Paganhill Inspiration, CD, TD). *Don Petrulis Photography*

174

immediately began exhibiting in both breed and obedience, and Speculation soon acquired both an American and Canadian championship and several obedience titles. She produced two champions, the most important being Ch. Pagan Hill Flower Child, UDT, a Group winner in Canada and dam of eleven champions. Flower was the foundation for Paganhill English Cockers.

Beth has bred nineteen champions to date. Among the better-known Paganhill English Cockers were Ch. Paganhill Bluenose; Ch. Pagan Hill Billy Blue Flash; Ch. Paganhill Commander In Chief, CD, an all-breed Best in Show winner; and Ch. Paganhill Persuasion, CDX, TD, WDX, who has a Highest Scoring Dog in Trial to his credit.

Persuasion, call-named "Powder," was Reserve Winners Dog from the 6–9 Puppy class at the 1982 ECSCA National Specialty. He completed his championship a year later and then entered the obedience ring, where he completed his CDX in three trials within four days. He was the second English Cocker to earn the new Junior Hunter title in April 1989, and he has two legs toward his Senior Hunter title. He is the sire of five champions to date.

With the purchase of Maidavale Trillium from Ann Eldredge in 1984, a parallel line has been added to Paganhill. Trillium has produced two champions so far. Ch. Paganhill Rambling Rose completed her title from the Puppy classes, and Ch. Paganhill Ultra Bright won the Sweepstakes at the Northern California Specialty in 1987.

Beth is a founding member of the Cascade English Cocker Spaniel Fanciers and has been either president or secretary of that club since 1976. She has been a member of the English Cocker Spaniel Club of America since 1968 and was elected as its president in 1989.

Barbara Murphy, Illinois: Daisymead

After involvement with several other larger breeds, Barbara decided to scale down in size, and on the advice of Kate Romanski contacted JoAnn Larsen Davis of Canterbury English Cockers. The result of that contact was a bitch puppy from a breeding of JoAnn's top producing Ch. Vari's Fascination and Ch. Dunelm Galaxy. That little puppy named Daisy grew up to become Ch. Canterbury's Razzle Dazzle, Barbara's very special introduction to English Cockers.

From a breeding to Ch. Kenobo Capricorn, Daisy produced the open marked tricolored dog Ch. Daisymead's Weekend Warrior. From her next litter, sired by Ch. Roundelay Rival, came Ch. Daisymead's Dilettante, a liver roan dog, and Ch. Daisymead's Blue Velvet. Blue

Velvet was then bred to Ch. Maidavale Firethorne and produced Barbara's first Group-placing homebred, Ch. Daisymead's Blue Ash.

From a breeding to Ch. Olde Spice Crusader and Blue Velvet came Barbara's second Group-placing dog, Ch. Daisymead's Dynasty, and his sisters, Ch. Daisymead's Roxy Music and Ch. Daisymead's Precious Moments. Dynasty has proven to be an excellent sire, and the Daisymead line remains strong through his offspring.

Barbara and John O'Brien, New Jersey: Mistral

Barbara and John acquired their first English Cocker in 1969. While she was a delightful companion, she was not up to the standard that they wanted. Fortunately, in 1970 they were able to import their foundation bitch, Ch. Leabank Love Affair, from Margaret Stevens in England.

Bred to both Ch. Dunelm Galaxy and Ch. Reklawholm Firebird, Love Affair produced seven champions, including Ch. Mistral Estragon, a top winning English Cocker owned and handled by Marge Bartelson.

While over the years John and Barbara have bred at least their share of champions, they are really most proud of the sound condition and stable temperament of these merry companions.

Nancy and Ed Overton, Texas

Nancy's introduction to the breed came in 1971 at the Great Barrington Club's Tracking Test, where she had gone with her two German Shepherds to compete. While there she saw Louise Shattuck handle Carry-On Crispin of El Paca, CDX, TD (later Ch. UDT) pass another Tracking Test.

Seven years later the memory of that day came back as she watched a Crispin granddaughter, Ch. Carry-On Chrysanthemum, CD (later UD), exhibited in obedience. She hurried home to buy her first puppy and ended up with two, Carry-On Pogety Possum and Carry-On Crazy Quilt.

These two proved easy learners whose obedience scores more than once tied for placements. Both girls went on to become champions and to earn CDX, TD and WDX titles in obedience and field.

Cathryn J. Pearce, Alaska: Ceridwen

Ch. Lochdene Straw Hat, a Scottish import, was purchased by Cathryn from Patricia Shaw of Lochdene Kennels. Straw Hat has

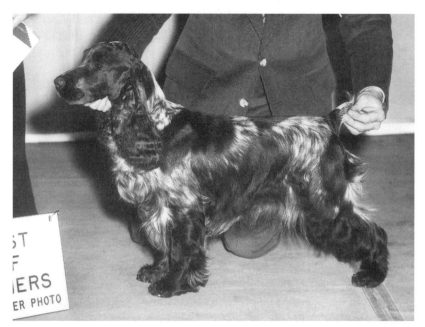

Ch. Leabank Love Affair, blue roan bitch (Ch. Leabank Luckstone ex Leabank Lovestory).
Evelyn M. Shafer

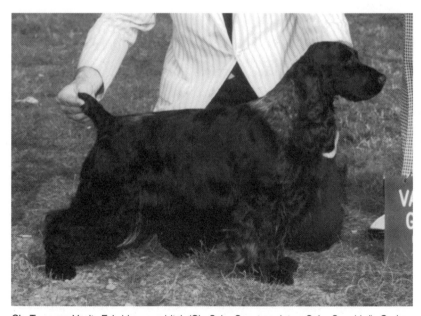

Ch. Trupence Vanity Fair, blue roan bitch (Ch. Soho Counterpoint ex Soho Songbird). *Graham*

177

several firsts to her credit. She is the first solid-colored English Cocker to attain her championship in Alaska, as well as the first English Cocker to learn a CD title there, which she did in her first three consecutive trials. Straw Hat is currently working on attaining her tracking title.

Kathleen Petruzzi, New Jersey: Carousel

Kathy acquired her first English Cocker from Mary Ann Alston in 1985, after having owned Great Danes for several years. This bitch, who finished easily, was Ch. Fieldstone Stardust Ruffles, a blue roan bitch, co-owned with Margaret Petruzzi. Ruffles was bred to Ch. Maidavale Night Flight, producing a champion male. She then bought a red bitch, Ch. Lorjos Fieldstone Nutmeg (Ch. Kavora Beau Regard ex Lorjos Something Sensational). Nutmeg took the Open Bitch Solid class at the 1987 National Specialty. She has been bred twice, and her second litter, by Ch. Hobbithill Ashwood Hi Class, produced two red bitches who were major pointed before they were one year old. Carousel Fieldstone Caress is owned by Mary Ann Alston and Mrs. Arthur Warner. Carousel Fieldstone Confec'n is owned by Kathy.

Kathy also owns Ch. Fieldstone Paint By Numbers, a blue roan and tan bitch (Ch. Ninebark Tarheel Major ex Ch. Fieldstone Maesgwyn Katrina), whose most recent litter is by Ch. Edgewood Play With Fire, whelped in July 1989.

Kathy is secretary of the Delaware Valley English Cocker Club.

Carolyn and Jesse Pfeiffer, Virginia: Trupence

Carolyn and Jesse became interested in English Cockers and showing dogs in 1967 through their teen-age daughter Bonnie, who had acquired a young roan male from Soho Kennels. This dog, Soho Peppercorn, was ably trained and piloted to a CD degree in three consecutive shows by Bonnie. It was then that Jesse decided to try his hand at showing the dog in the conformation ring. As luck would have it, Jesse showed him to a major point win in his very first attempt at handling. When Peppercorn went Best of Winners at the 1970 English Cocker Spaniel Club of America National Specialty, Carolyn and Jesse were really hooked on the sport.

Their interest in breeding began after the acquisition of Soho Aperitif, a Mother's Day present for Carolyn. After completing her championship, Aperitif was bred to Ch. Soho Star Rover and produced the beginning of a long line of Trupence champions, Ch. Trupence Naughty Marietta and Ch. Trupence My Fair Lady.

Certain dogs come to mind whenever Carolyn and Jesse review their involvement with English Cockers. Ch. Trupence Vanity Fair, WD, was an excellent show dog, winning multiple Sporting Group placements, and a good brood bitch, producing several champions that exhibited her outstanding attributes. She worked well in the field and was a loving companion.

Vanity Fair's daughter, Am. & Can. Ch. Trupence Girl Friday, also comes to mind. Although not campaigned as a champion, she excelled as a brood bitch. Two of her most important get are Am. & Can. Ch. Trupence Friday's Child and Ch. Trupence Fife and Drum. Friday's Child won many Bests of Breed and Group placements in both the United States and Canada. Although used only sparingly as a stud, he produced several champions both for Trupence and other kennels.

Finally, there is Ch. Trupence Fife and Drum, a strikingly handsome and aristocratic blue roan dog, who passed on his many virtues to his offspring, many of whom earned championships. He is listed as an ECSCA top producer.

Ch. Trupence Maid Marian of Maro is one of Trupence's most recent champions. Sired by Aro's Pam Pam, she is a good example of the kind of English Cocker Carolyn and Jesse strive to breed.

Over thirty-two homebred champions later, Carolyn and Jesse state the secret to their success is tenacity and perseverance, attention to detail and the eye of an artist.

Eugene Phoa, Edmonton, Canada: Wittersham

The Wittersham English Cockers began in 1959 with the purchase of a red bitch in Australia largely of Treetops breeding. Although she eventually proved to be a nonproducer, her temperament was such that she made Eugene Phoa a fan of this breed for life. He chose the prefix "Wittersham" purely because that was the name of the family home in Singapore where he was then residing.

The first Wittersham show-quality English Cocker also came from Australia from the Yunbeai (an Australian aboriginal word meaning "animal spirit") Kennels of Mr. and Mrs. Gooding. That dog, a red male, had already completed his Australian title and had won four all-breed Bests in Show in Australia. He was subsequently shown in Malaysia and Singapore under the name of Ch. Yunbeai Sea Captain of Wittersham. He was a grandson of the great English Show Ch. Collinwood Silver Lariot. When Sea Captain was bred to the black bitch Ch. Yunbeai Kismet of Wittersham, another acquisition from the Goodings, the foundation of Wittersham was begun.

In the early 1970s Eugene purchased English Show Ch. Valsissimo of Misbourne of Wittersham from D. M. Hahn. This dog was sired by Sunglint of Sorbrook, one of the most significant red sires of modern times. Valsissimo has undoubtably had more influence to date on the Wittershams than any other dog. He proved to be one of those dogs which could be linebred very closely without any harmful effects. By taking advantage of this attribute, another string of winners was produced.

One of the most important results of these linebreedings on Valsissimo is Am. & Can. Ch. Wittersham's Emblem. Emblem's show career includes thirteen all-breed Bests in Show in Canada, as well as multiple Groups in the United States. Emblem was the top English Cocker for two years in Canada and for one year in the United States.

In 1976 Eugene and the Wittersham Cockers moved to Canada, and since 1979 the showing side of operations has been almost exclusively under the guidance of Barbara Heckerman of Wyncrest Kennels. Under her capable hands the Wittersham Cockers have done very well, particularly at Specialties.

Some of the more famous Wittershams include Am. & Can. Ch. Wittersham's Mythical Galateia, Best of Winners at an English Cocker Club of America National Specialty; Am. & Can. Ch. Wittersham's Debutante, with two all-breed Canadian Bests in Show, claimed as the top winning bitch of the breed in Canadian history; Am. & Can. Ch. Wittersham's Wyncrest Lovesong, Best-In-Sweepstakes at an English Cocker Club of America National Specialty; Am. & Can. Ch. Wittersham's Charlemagne, Winners Dog at both the Canadian and American National Specialties; and Am. & Can. Ch. Wittersham's Rhiannon, Best of Breed at the first Canadian National Specialty.

Also closely associated with Wittersham are two dogs whose influence on the breed has yet to be settled. These two dogs, both imported from England, are English Show Ch. and Am. & Can. Ch. Bryansbrook High Society and English Show Ch. Misbourne Postmark, both of whom unfortunately died before reaching old age. High Society, who had taken Best of Breed at the prestigious Crufts Dog Show in England, has consistently passed on his beautiful head and eye to his many offspring. Progeny from both High Society and Postmark are just now achieving high honors in the show ring.

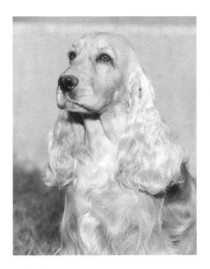

Am. & Can. Ch. Wittersham's Rhiannon, red bitch (Eng., Am. & Can. Ch. Bryansbrook High Society ex Can. Ch. Wittersham's Bonnie Noelle). *Mikron Photos Ltd.*

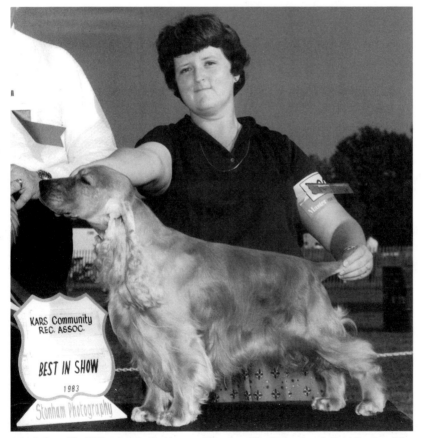

Am. & Can. Ch. Wittersham's Emblem, golden dog (Ch. Wittersham's Bon Gout ex Glen Astrid Morar of Wittersham). *Stonham Photography*

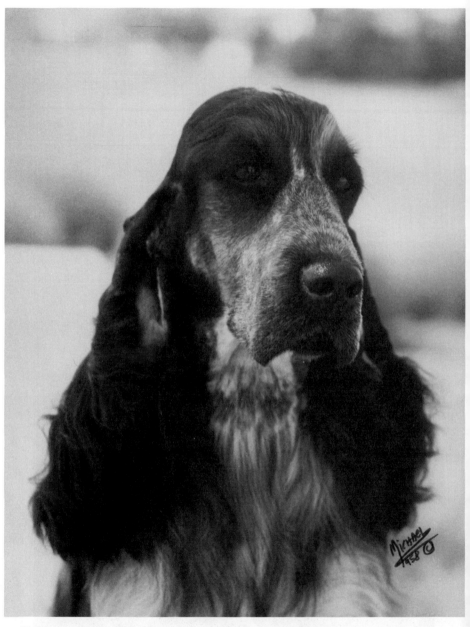

Ch. Pineshire's Star 'N Wyncastle, TD, WDX, blue roan and tan bitch (Ch. Kenobo Capricorn ex Ch. Kenobo Spark of Magic).

Michael © 1958

Nancy Praiswater, California: Star-Vue

Star-Vue English Cockers began with the purchase of two Ch. Kenobo Capricorn daughters. In the early days Star-Vue and Wyncastle co-owned their foundation bitches and co-bred their first litters. The first daughter, Ch. Pineshire's Star'N Wyncastle, bred by Yolanda Brancato, arrived in December of 1974 and was dubbed "Josie." Her show career was short but successful. She completed her championship at eight months of age with four major wins.

Her first litter, by Ch. Graecroft Tarus of Wyncastle, produced a single puppy and her only champion. This puppy, also a blue roan and tan, became Ch. Wyncastle Momento of Star-Vue, who in turn produced numerous champions for Star-Vue. Josie's last litter, sired by Ch. Mourning Dove Jacob of Star-Vue, WDX, produced another single puppy, Star-Vue's Xanadu. This bitch in turn is the dam of two champions to date, Ch. Star-Vue Celebrates Sonrise and Ch. Star-Vue'N Silverline Rejoice. Both of these Star-Vue Cockers were sired by Ch. Woodlea Dicroft Patriot.

The second Ch. Kenobo Capricorn daughter to arrive was Ch. Graecroft Legend of Wyn-Star. "Dolly," as she was called, was an excellent producer with over eight champions to her credit. From her first litter, sired by Ch. Carachelle Crockett, came the black and white bitch Ch. Star-Vue's Trix E of Wyncastle. "Trixie" produced a lovely black and white male, Ch. Star-Vue's Hat Trix, now co-owned with Star-Vue by Jane Doty of Graecroft Kennels, and sired by the liver and white dog Ch. Springfield Michelob, CD.

Nancy and Star-Vue have now entered into their fourth generation of champions from their two Capricorn daughters, Josie and Dolly. The culmination of both foundation bitches is found in the chocolate and white bitch Star-Vue's Fudgie Brown, who is just starting her show career.

Nancy's advice to newcomers in the breed is to watch, wait and study before purchasing a dog. Good advice to everyone purchasing a dog, whether for the first time or the tenth time.

Carol Richter, Washington: Topsham

As an exhibitor and breeder, Carol has been most interested in the overall versatility of the breed. She has been involved in English Cockers since 1975 and has been an active member of the English Cocker Club of America.

Her first bitch, Ch. Kenobo My Blue Heaven, CD, TD, WD,

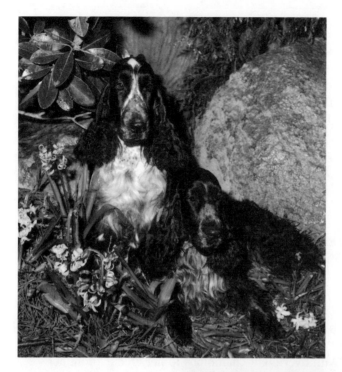

Ch. Topsham's Smoke N' Ash, CD, TD, JH, WDX *(left)*, blue roan dog, with Topsham's Sky High, blue roan bitch (Ch. Somerset's Sky Pilot ex Ch. Kenobo My Blue Heaven, CD, TD, WD).

Michael Allen

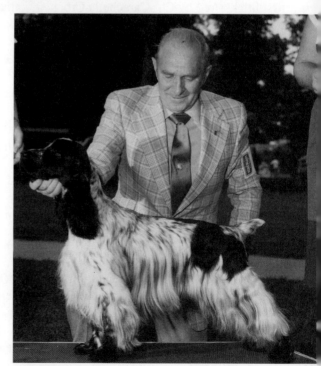

Ch. Rick N Pat's Simply Classic, blue roan dog (Ch. Winsonem's Windstar Major ex Ch. Rick N Pat's Custom Made).

Missy Yuhl

184

bred by Helga Tustin, is the dam of six offspring holding Tracking titles. Ch. Topsham's Smoke N' Ash, CD, TD, WDX, is the most impressive of her offspring. He earned his CD in both the United States and Canada, quickly followed by his TD and seven WDXs! He is a steady field dog, holding his own in trials with field-bred Springers.

Carol bought a liver roan bitch, Ch. Amawalk's Darkenwald Bettina, CD, TD, WD, which produced two litters. Carol breeds infrequently and starts all of her puppies on birds. She is interested in placing puppies in good obedience homes as well as show homes.

She also owned the National Specialty Sweepstakes Winner, Ch. Maidavale William of Orange, CD.

Pat and Rick Rickford, Utah: Rick N Pat

Rick and Pat's interest in the breed began in 1947 when they purchased several English Cockers from Laura Clark of Quarto K Kennels. From Laddie Carswell they purchased Philsworth's Mollie O'Laddie and bred her to Philsworth's Sir Cedric. This breeding produced Ch. Dustie Lou O'Laddie, their foundation bitch.

The first big show thrill for Pat and Rick came with a dog they also purchased from Laddie Carswell, Ch. Dandy of Ranch-Aero, who went Best in Show at the Colorado Kennel Club. Next came an English import, Ch. Courtdale Crown Regent. "Andy," as he was called, was bred to Ch. Dustie Lou O'Laddie and produced the first Cocker to carry their prefix, Ch. Rick and Pat's Bleu Boy. Bleu Boy was a multiple-Group winner and the sire of five champions.

Although Rick and Pat have bred very sparingly over the years, their English Cockers have consistently placed in the Group, and many have attained their championships.

Among their many accomplishments, Ch. Rick N Pat's New Look was honored as a top producer in 1975 and 1976. Ch. Rick N Pat's Custom Made, a Group-winning bitch, was in the top rankings of the breed from 1977 through 1979.

Ruston and Linda Robinson, Georgia: Rustlin

The Robinsons' involvement with the breed began in 1976 with the acquisition of Merryborne Sesame, a two-year-old red bitch. She in turn was bred to Charlton's Tar and Feathers to produce the first Rustlin puppies. Among this first litter were Am. & Can. Ch. Rustlin Gallant MacDuff, co-bred with Jo Ella Young; Am. & Can. Ch. Rustlin

Valiant Rugby, CD; and Ch. Caib Chelsea of Rustlin, herself a top producer.

Am. & Can. Ch. Rustlin Gallant MacDuff was one of the few solid black dogs to achieve a Best in Show, and this he accomplished twice during his show career. His show career ended with ninety-five Best of Breed wins and twenty-five Group placements. He is the sire of seven champions, including Ch. Diplomat So Much Velvet, a top-ranked English Cocker in 1982. He was and will always be a very special dog to Ruston and Linda and his many friends.

Ch. Rustlin Puttin on the Ritz, UDT, was a top-ranked obedience dog in 1986 and 1987. Ch. Rustlin's Dauntless Diplomat and Ch. Rustlin Windsong Golden Bear have also excelled in the show ring with multiple Group wins and placements.

Lisa M. Ross, Virginia: Winfree

After showing Irish Setters in both conformation and obedience for many years, Lisa acquired her first English Cocker, Maidavale Mariner, from Ted and Ann Eldredge. Next to join the family was Spoutspring Gentle One. "Genie," as she was called, became the foundation bitch of Winfree and was the top producing bitch in 1987 with six champions and numerous other pointed get to her credit.

The first dog to carry the Winfree prefix was sired by Maidavale Mariner out of Soho Precisely. This dog, Winfree Little Rascal, turned out to be something quite special. He finished in thirteen shows, went Best of Breed over specials three times, and was just fifteen months old when he attained his championship. Since then, in very limited showing, he has amassed many Bests of Breed, a Group I, and numerous other Group placements. He also has several champion children to his credit.

The first litter bred by Winfree was sired by Ch. Maidavale Firethorne out of Spoutspring Gentle One. This litter of four produced two champions, Winfree's Firefall and Winfree's Wildfire, CD.

Six more litters have been bred by Lisa since then, and all have added success to the Winfree name. Ch. Winfree Caped Crusader and Ch. Winfree's C-Witch, sired by Ch. Olde Spice Crusader and Spoutspring Gentle One, are from Lisa's fourth litter.

Connie Sabroske, Florida: Beowulf

Connie Sabroske acquired her first English Cocker, Beowulf's Dwana, from the Gala Glen Kennels of Pat Gallagher. Due to her

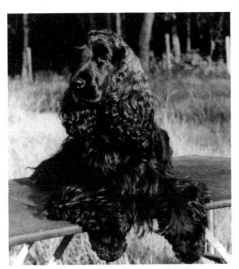

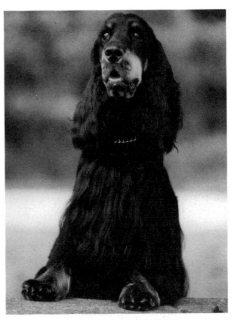

Am. & Can. Ch. Rustlin Gallant MacDuff, black dog (Charlton's Tar and Feathers ex Merryborne Sesame).

Ch. Rustlin Puttin on the Ritz, UDT, black and tan dog (Ch. Glenmora Diplomat in Brass ex Stonehenge Satin Doll).

Ch. Rustlin Windsong's Golden Bear, red dog (Ch. Rustlin Dauntless Diplomat ex Rustlin Gone with the Wind).

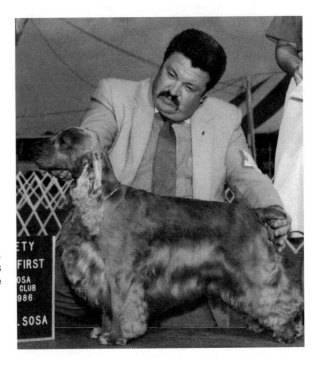

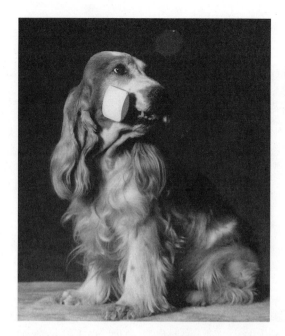

Coltrim Cream Tea, CDX, TD, orange roan bitch (Seltaeb Prince of Orange ex Coltrim Carolina Moon).

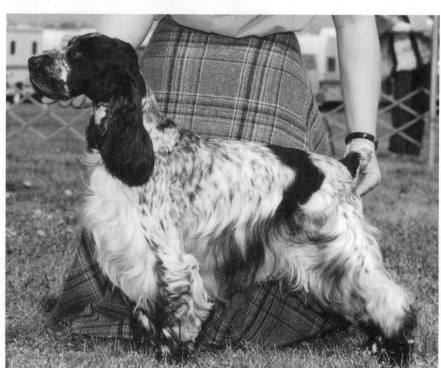

Ch. Winfree Little Rascal, blue roan dog (Ch. Maidavale Mariner ex Soho Precisely).

Bernard W. Kernan

aversion to the show ring, Dwana never completed her championship but instead proved her worth to Connie by presenting her with five puppies sired by Ch. Somerset's Blue Omega. One of these pups, Ch. Beowulf's King Arthur, became Connie's first homebred champion by attaining his title in eight weeks. Dwana's second litter, by Ch. Dunelm Guardsman, produced Ch. Beowulf Misty Stone of Scone, owned by Jean Goldstein.

Connie obtained her second bitch, Tarheel Caroline of Beowulf, from the Teals as a ten-week-old puppy. By the age of ten months she had accumulated fourteen points, including a four-point major win. Caroline completed her championship under the guidance of Gary Engle, her handler, and finished 1986 as a top ten–ranked English Cocker bitch. Caroline has produced several litters for Beowulf and is considered by Connie to be her foundation bitch.

Mary J. Sharpe-Harkins, California: Shaemar

Mary Sharpe-Harkins acquired her first English Cocker from Donna Palmer (Do-Bain) and Judith Frank (Wedgewood) in 1979. This Cocker, Am. & Can. Ch. Do-Bain Happy Time Gal, was entirely owner handled to her championship and was the Best of Opposite Sex winner at the 1982 English Cocker Spaniel Club of America National Specialty. She completed 1982 as the sixth-ranked English Cocker bitch with several Best of Breed wins at supported and all-breed shows. She is the dam of three champions.

Happy Time Gal was bred twice. The result of the first breeding, to Ch. Kenobo Rabbit of Nadou, was three puppies, of which two acquired their championships. These two cockers, Ch. Shaemar's Happy Tan Shoes and Ch. Shaemar's Happy Tale, were both Specialty winners in 1984.

Bred a second time, to Ch. Olde Spice Crusader, Happy Time Gal produced Ch. Shaemar's Suzy Creamcheese, who won a five-point major from breeder and judge Anne Rogers Clark.

The next generation at Shaemar has also been very successful. Ch. Shaemar's Happy Tale has produced one champion each from her litters sired by Ch. Wyncastle's Lookin at You Kid and Ch. Wyncastle's Blu Magician. Ch. Shaemar's Darn Tootin' is co-owned with Kay and Robert Sutter (Stardust). Ch. Shaemar's Dustruffle was Best in Sweeps and Winners Bitch from the Bred by Exhibitor class at the Cascade English Cocker Specialty in August 1987. Both of these dogs finished in 1987, making Happy Tale, like her dam, a top producer for that year.

Also of much pride to Shaemar are Ch. Shaemar Timmara Fyrebrand (bred in association with Pam Dahl of Timmara Kennels), who finished at twelve months of age; and Carra-Lee Firenza O'Timmara, who went Best of Winners and Best of Opposite Sex at the English Cocker Spaniel Club of Northern California's first Specialty.

Louise Shattuck, Massachusetts: Carry-On

Louise Shattuck began in English Cockers about 1945, although she had owned American Cockers before that time. She has been breeding sound, working dogs concentrating on two lines. Her orange line is descended from Coltrim Cream Tea, CDX, TD, an English import, and her blue line is descended from Ch. Carry-On Crispin of El Paca, UDT. Crispin was the first UDT champion in the breed in the United States.

To date Louise has bred fifteen champions, most of which are titled in obedience, tracking, and working. She has achieved fifty-nine obedience and tracking titles! She does not participate in the Working Dog tests, as she does not like to kill birds, but many dogs of her breeding have attained their Working Dog titles.

In addition to her extensive activities with her dogs, Louise is an accomplished writer and artist. She is the author of two published books, and her animal sculptures in bronze are prized by collectors. She also is a great illustrator and cartoonist. Her drawings appear frequently in magazines, and she has been called upon to supply trophies for many English Cocker Specialty shows.

Faith and Ken Sizemore, Virginia: Encore

Encore is based on both Gunpowder and Sunspan lines. Faith and Ken's foundation dog is Ch. Gunpowder Encore of Sunspan, who has proven to be a sire and grandsire of worth for Encore.

The foundation bitch at Encore is Ch. Sunspan Southern Style, a Group-placing daughter sired by Ch. Olde Spice Crusader. Five of her offspring have finished, including Ch. Sunspan Silver Sovereign, and Ch. Sunspan Rave Reviews.

Merry temperament, sound bodies and multifaceted talent are the most important breeding goals at Encore.

190

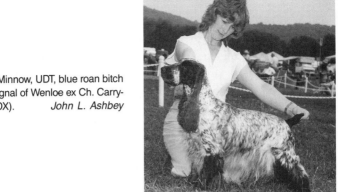

Ch. Carry-On Catch A Minnow, UDT, blue roan bitch (Ch. Dunelm Smoke Signal of Wenloe ex Ch. Carry-On Rackety Coon, CDX).   *John L. Ashbey*

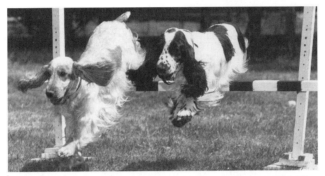

Ch. Carry-On Gopher Baroque, CDX, TD *(left)*, orange roan bitch (The Town Crier ex Carry-On Cornflakes), with Ch. Carry-On Badger, UDT, black and white bitch (Ch. Braeside Donegal Tweed ex Carry-On Gopher Baroque, CDX, TD).

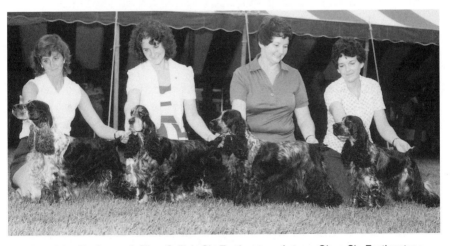

Left to right: Ch. Graecroft Silver Solitair, Ch. Featherstone Autumn Glory, Ch. Featherstone Sneak Preview and Ch. Featherstone Autumn Review.

Carolyn Sisson, California: Prima

Carolyn's first love and interest in the English Cocker was the direct result of her association with a beautiful blue roan dog named Ch. Ancram's Paul. The first English Cocker to come to Prima was a Paul daughter named Serr'a April Fantasy. She in turn was bred to Ch. Ancram's William, giving Carolyn her first Prima English Cocker champion, Prima's Pixie Paula of Sha Ray.

A second Paul daughter, Ch. Legionaire By Golly Miss Molly, was bred to Ch. Ancram's Desert Sheik and produced the black dog Ch. Prima's Ace of Spades, CD, PC (Mexican CD).

Prima has also produced Ch. Prima's Lucabuc Cowboy, a black and tan dog, and Ch. Prima's Sir Winston, an orange roan dog.

Anna E. Skomp, Nevada: Copperclad

Anna Skomp has owned English Cockers for twenty-three years; her preference is for solids. Her first dog was purchased from Lynn Clark's Soho Kennels when Anna was only ten years old. She showed this red bitch, Ch. Soho Copper Primrose, CD, entirely herself, was only twelve years old when she finished Posey's championship and her obedience degree.

When Lynn Clark decided to concentrate on particolors, Anna and her mother acquired additional Soho dogs, whom they bred to some Merryborne imports in the 1970s. In 1972 they bought Ch. Merryborne Hallmark and bred him to their red bitch, Ch. Merryborne Copperclad. This breeding produced Ch. Copperclad Tubby Essington, who was later sold to Ralph Huber in Ohio.

Anna's lines, through the Merryborne dogs, are behind many of the Fireside, Canterbury and Briarpatch solid English Cockers. She continues to show and breed occasionally. Her latest entry is a black bitch, Merryborne Simonetta; and she has bred Tylerthyme Copperclad Melo D, a red bitch, to Ch. Merryborne Superstar, who is a younger brother to Ch. Merryborne Copperclad. She hopes to retain the quality of the original English imports through this combination.

Terry Jo and Sandra J. Smith, Massachusetts: Featherstone

A search for the right breed, a breed that was active, small and compatible with all the other animals in the home (goats, steers, rabbits, and cats) led to a phone call to Jane Doty of Graecroft Kennels. An invitation to Graecroft resulted in love at first sight with Poppy, a four-month-old blue roan puppy who came to live with Terry Jo. Poppy was to become Ch. Graecroft Silver Solitaire.

Poppy was bred to Ch. Kenobo Confetti. The lone survivor from that litter, a blue roan and tan bitch, became Ch. Featherstone Autumn Glory, and Featherstone English Cockers was born. Autumn Glory, or "Abby," in turn has produced two champions, Ch. Featherstone Sneak Preview and Ch. Featherstone Autumn Review. Both of these girls were sired by Ch. Somerset's Stage Door Review.

Vicky Spice, Wisconsin: Olde Spice

As a child, Vicky had always dreamed of owning a show dog. As a teen-ager that dream came true in a little blue roan puppy obtained from Cindy Baumeister and Diane Dambeck of Cindione Kennels. That puppy grew up to be Ch. Cindione Andrea Christine, CD, WDX ("Christy"), and the dream became a reality.

In order to begin a breeding program, Vicky purchased a young blue roan male from Carachelle Kennels. This dog, Carachelle Court Jester, completed his championship very quickly and was bred to Christy. The result was three males, all of which finished their championships by the time they were eighteen months of age. The first of these males, Ch. Olde Spice Anchors Away, is owned by Lynn Sharkey; the second, Ch. Olde Spice Buccaneer, is owned by Jan Peterson; and the third male, who became Ch. Olde Spice Crusader, is owned by Vicky and has attained the most impressive record of the three.

Crusader obtained his championship in seven shows. Shown as a champion he obtained multiple Group wins and received three National Specialty Awards of Merit. In addition, he has proven his worth as a sire, with thirty-seven champions to his credit, and many more pointed offspring near their titles. Among his offspring are multiple Specialty and all-breed Best in Show winners, both in the United States and in Canada.

One of Crusader's most notable children is Ch. Olde Spice Sailors Beware ("Dusty"). At the tender age of six months and three days, Dusty attended her first AKC show and promptly went Best of Breed over seven champions, including her sire. Dusty provided Vicky with her biggest thrill when she completed her championship at thirteen months of age at the English Cocker Spaniel Club of America National Specialty by going Winners Bitch, Best of Winners and Best Bred by Exhibitor. Her show career certainly fulfilled Vicky's childhood dream

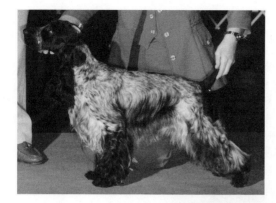

Ch. Cindione Andrea Christine, CD, WDX, blue roan bitch (Ch. Carachelle Casino ex Soho Refrain). *Lloyd W. Olson Studio*

Ch. Carachelle Court Jester, blue roan dog (Ch. Ranzfel Newsflash, Am. & Can. TD, ex Ch. Carachelle Coquette). *Ralph Karlen*

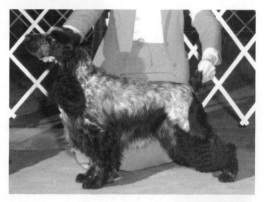

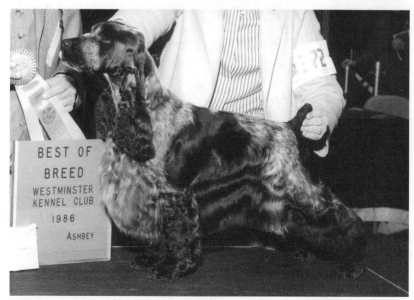

Ch. Olde Spice Sailors Beware, blue roan bitch (Ch. Olde Spice Crusader ex Windswept's Katherine). *Ashbey Photography*

of owning a show dog. She has won an unprecedented three National Specialties with her latest win occurring in June 1989, three all-breed Bests in Show, twenty Group I, and over forty other Group placements en route to becoming the top winning bitch in breed history, completely owner handled by Vicky.

Barbara and Walter B. Steward, Michigan: Askonandy Farm

Walt and Barb have been involved with English Cockers since 1982, when they purchased their foundation bitch, Ch. Springfield Indian Summer, Am. & Can. TD.

The second addition to the household was Do-Bain's Windjammer, Am. & Can. CD, TDX, Can. TD. Jamie turned out to be a natural, enthusiastic tracker and retriever. The result of a breeding of these two excellent trackers produced Askonandy Serendipity, Am. & Can. TD, and Ch. Askonandy Holiday Sailor, TDX, Can. TD, the first homebred champion for Askonandy.

Walt and Barb are just now starting their third generation of tracking English Cockers and have hopes that young Askonandy's Rum Runner will follow in his grandsire and uncle's pawprints.

Nancy and Brad Sweet, Minnesota: Sweet Apple

Sweet Apple began in 1980 with the acquisition of two English Cockers from Donna Kovar's Ashgrove Kennel, Ashgrove Alistair Blue, CD, and Ch. Ashgrove Abigail Blue. Abby was to make a most significant mark for Sweet Apple by producing two of the nation's top bitches, Ch. Sweet Apple Granny Smith and Ch. Sweet Apple Beacon.

Granny Smith's soundness, style and enthusiasm for showing, combined with Bob and Delores Burkholder's superb handling, proved to be a winning combination that resulted in a remarkable show career. Granny Smith won Groups in each of five consecutive years, during which she also took a turn in the whelping box. Granny Smith became the top English Cocker bitch in the country for 1983 and 1985. In 1984, while on maternity leave, she relinquished the top spot to her litter sister, Ch. Sweet Apple Beacon.

From Granny Smith's first litter came Ch. Sweet Apple Wellington, a Group winner and a proven producer of champions himself. Granny Smith's second litter produced Ch. Sweet Apple Gala and Ch. Sweet Apple Ben Davis. Ben provided Brad and Nancy with quite a thrill when he won Best in Sweepstakes at the 1988 English Cocker

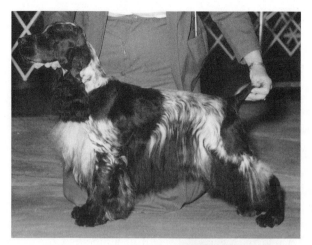

Ch. Sweet Apple Wellington, blue roan dog (Ch. Applewyn Argyle ex Ch. Sweet Apple Granny Smith).
Booth Photo

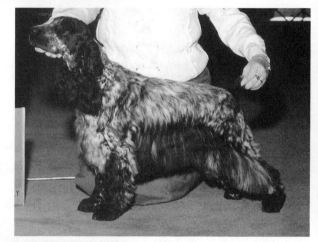

Ch. Stardust Crystal Gayle, blue roan bitch (Ch. Edgewood Incumbent ex Ch. Stardust Diamond Lil).
Ashbey Photography

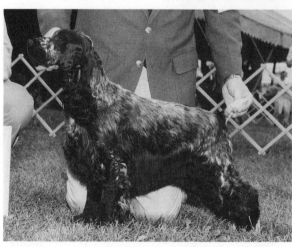

Ch. Edgewood Incumbent, blue roan dog (Ch. Edgewood Fan-Tan ex Kenobo Edgewood Eureka).
John L. Ashbey

Club of America National Specialty. Granny Smith has also produced another star for Nancy and Brad, Ch. Sweet Apple Cecilia. Cecilia, a blue roan bitch, was sired by Ch. Reklawholm Rockbeat.

Not to be outdone by her beautiful daughters, Ch. Ashgrove Abigail Blue came out of retirement to win the Veteran Bitch class at the 1987 National Specialty show.

Susan Thompson, South Carolina: Solivia

Solivia English Cockers had its beginning in 1973 with the purchase of Merry Mist Magic O'Merrybuck from Joyce Thomas. She was sired by Ch. Duke of Diamonds, and her dam was Int. Ch. On Time Lucy's Merry Mist Bea.

Several years and several career moves later, Susan obtained a black and white puppy from Natalie Lane. This puppy was to become Ch. Fayrplace Far Star of Solivia, the sire of four champions himself. One of these four, Ch. Jaclyn Summer Magic O'Solivia, finished at just over a year with five major wins.

Solivia has also produced Ch. Solivia Magic Memories and Ch. Solivia Foxfyre Fantasia, and is home to the Group-winning bitch Ch. Stardust Crystal Gayle.

Bonnie and Mark Threlfall, Pennsylvania: Edgewood

Bonnie's partnership with Helga Tustin spans many years and includes many great dogs. Bonnie co-owned her first English Cocker with Helga Tustin approximately twenty years ago. Ch. Kenobo Blue Astro, CDX, was his name, and his most notable claim to fame was capturing Best in Sweepstakes at the 1969 English Cocker National Specialty. Then came Robby, and from Robby, Goat.

Robby, who was otherwise known as Ch. Kenobo Rabbit of Nadou, was ranked as the number one English Cocker in 1972 and 1973 and placed three times in the Sporting group at the Westminster Kennel Club show. His show record was enviable, but his true strength was as a sire. His offspring include fifty-five champions, four all-breed Best in Show winners, two National Specialty winners, five top producers, eight obedience titleholders, and Goat.

Ch. Kenobo Capricorn, or "Goat," as he was known by all, was a multiple Specialty and Best in Show winner and was the top English Cocker in 1974 and 1975. He won the English Cocker National Specialty twice, the latter being a most memorable win from the Veteran class in 1982.

Inheriting his prepotent traits from his grandfather, Ch. Dunelm Galaxy, and his father, Goat was the sire of 119 champions including 2 all-breed AKC Best in Show winners; 2 all-breed Canadian Best in Show winners; 6 top producers; 4 National Specialty winners; 21 obedience titleists; and 8 English Cockers with Working Certificates. Both Robby and Goat were bred by and co-owned with Helga Tustin of Kenobo Kennels.

During that early period, Bonnie acquired a blue roan bitch named Graecroft Calliope. This bitch, whose unusual call name was "Crow," completed her championship easily. Some of her notable wins include Winners Bitch at the 1975 National Specialty at the age of six months, and Best of Opposite Sex at the 1978 National Specialty.

However, her most notable accomplishments were achieved in the whelping box. She was bred four times and produced nine champions. She is the foundation upon which Edgewood is built. From her first litter to Ch. Surrey Blue Stone came Ch. Edgewood Turquoise, who in turn produced Ch. Edgewood Decapo. From her second litter of five, sired by Ch. Kenobo Oliver Luv, four finished their championships. These include Ch. Edgewood Liberty Valence and Ch. Kenobo Amana of Edgewood, who in turn produced Ch. Kenobo Edgewood Eureka, herself the dam of six champions to date. Calliope was bred a third time to Ch. Reklawholm Firebird and produced Ch. Edgewood Excalibur and Ch. Edgewood Play With Fire. Her last litter, sired by Ch. Kenobo Capricorn, yielded Ch. Edgewood Fan-Tan.

Due to their rigorous and time-consuming schedule as all-breed professional handlers, Mark and Bonnie limit their breeding activities to approximately one litter a year.

Katherine Touhey, Minnesota

Katherine purchased her first English Cocker from Roz Schneider of Tradewind Kennels in 1980. This bitch, Tradewind's Tatiana, was bred to Ch. Stardust Silver Dollar and produced Katherine's first home-bred and Group-winning champion, Ch. Little River's Gabrielle. Gabrielle has the honor of being one of the youngest English Cockers to win a Sporting Group, being just ten months old when she accomplished this.

Helga Tustin, Mississippi: Kenobo

Kenobo is a name so intertwined with English Cockers in the United States that it has influenced almost every line in existence today.

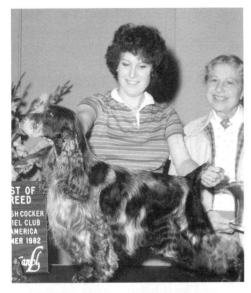

Ch. Kenobo Capricorn, blue roan dog (Ch. Kenobo Rabbit of Nadou ex Ch. Kenobo Silver Charm).
Carl Lindemaier

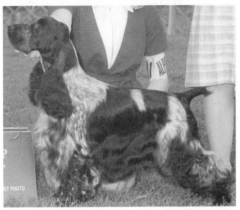

Ch. Kenobo Rabbit of Nadou, blue roan dog (Ch. Dunelm Galaxy ex Ch. Cygnet's Raspberry, CD).

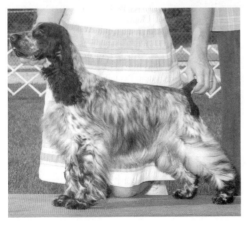

Ch. Little River's Gabrielle, blue roan bitch (Ch. Stardust Silver Dollar ex Tradewind's Tatiana).
Martin Booth

Combined with Dunelm, the two names are synonymous with English Cocker Spaniels in America.

Helga Tustin first saw an English Cocker when she was living in a New York apartment in the 1940s. In 1949 she purchased a tricolored male, Surrey Triumphant, from Olga Rogers. Through him, Helga became interested in obedience and eventually began to show in obedience trials and received her first exposure to dog shows. It was love at first sight, and through the tutorship of Seymour and Maurie Prager, Helga acquired her first show dogs. The first Kenobo litter was from Ch. On Time Suzanne's Major Rufus and Colinwood Silver Bangle, a black and white bitch imported by Helga. Ch. Kenobo Blithe Spirit, an orange roan, the first of more than fifty Kenobo champions, came from that litter.

The Kenobo-Dunelm combination came about when Helga first saw Ch. Dunelm Galaxy. To her, he was the epitome of the English Cocker both in temperament and conformation. She bred various bitches to him, a total of thirteen times, and he is behind her greatest dogs.

The first bitch she bred to Galaxy was Ch. Kenobo Moonlight Majic (Ch. Silver Lariot of Strathpine ex Ch. Cygnet's Raspberry). Raspberry was owned by Nancy Swan, and on condition that she be bred to Lariot, Helga was able to buy her. From that breeding came one of the breed's top producing bitches, Majic. From that first litter to Galaxy came Ch. Kenobo Constellation and Ch. Kenobo Blue Astro, CDX, who was owned by Bonnie Proctor (Threlfall) and eventually by Scott Proctor. The mating of Galaxy and Majic was repeated three times and produced a total of fourteen champions.

Constellation was the dog that most closely approximated the type Helga has strived for at Kenobo, although he was sold to Pam Hall as a puppy and achieved his winning record, including two Bests in Show, five Specialty Best of Breed wins and forty-nine Group placements, under her guidance. He was the sire of thirty-six champions.

Helga considers the best bitch she has bred to be Ch. Kenobo Silver Charm, a blue roan sired by Ch. Kenobo Oliver Luv and out of Ch. Kenobo Charm Bracelet. Her claim to fame in the whelping box comes from her mating to Ch. Kenobo Rabbit of Nadou to produce Ch. Kenobo Capricorn.

Rabbit is the son of Ch. Dunelm Galaxy bred to Ch. Cygnet's Raspberry. He was whelped in 1973 and sold as a puppy to Mrs. Dan Roth in Illinois. He finished his championship at just over one year of age and was spotted a year later by Bonnie Threlfall. She persuaded

Helga to buy him back, and upon his return he was co-owned and handled by Bonnie throughout his show and stud career. Among his illustrious offspring was the great Ch. Kenobo Capricorn, leading sire in the history of the breed and a top contender in the show ring during a long and successful career.

According to Helga, in choosing a puppy, the most important consideration is temperament. The English Cocker must be an outgoing, happy, agreeable dog, able to adapt to all situations. Early socialization is a must in her prescription for producing good dispositions, and all her puppies over the years have received a great deal of attention from the time they are able to walk. She is particular about homes for her puppies and discourages those dogs she considers pets from being bred.

Although Helga has curtailed her breeding program in the past few years, she maintains her interest in the breed, and in 1989 a young puppy, Skylark's Pumpkin of Kenobo, though not bred by her, was entered at the American Spaniel Club show—and has since completed her championship, by the age of thirteen months.

Susie Vallier, Texas: Reverie

After a few years of breeding Irish Setters, Susie felt a need for a smaller dog but one that would be compatible with her Irish. The English Cocker fulfilled that need, and in 1978 Susie's first English Cocker came to live at Reverie. That first dog was to become Ch. Inglenook Indigo Bunting.

A year later Susie requested a bitch from Georgia Brown from a breeding of Ch. Connemara Sweet Charity to Ch. Maidavale Firethorne. The result of that request was Brownhaven Reverie A L'Orange. "Lori," as she was called, capped her quest for her championship with a five-point major win at the Fort Worth show.

Next for Lori came her very productive career as a mother. Bred the first time to Ch. Wingslade Ringmaster, she produced four champions, including Ch. Reverie Just Bidin' My Time, a blue roan bitch owned by Corey McLean; Ch. Reverie Ange D'Or, an orange bitch owned by Doug Shelton; Ch. Reverie Hello Dolly, a blue roan bitch owned by Billy Abraham; and Ch. Reverie Extraordinaire, a blue roan and tan dog owned by Susie. Leased to Betsy Wahlberg for her second breeding, Lori produced four more champions, including Ch. Cambridge Little Blu Audrey and Ch. Cambridge Ariel Stoutheart. This litter was sired by Ch. Stardust Silver Dollar.

To date Lori has produced nine champions, with several other pointed sons and daughters well on their way to their championships. Lori's latest champion is Gentree Reverie Vieux Carré, a black and white ticked bitch sired by Ch. Edgewood Fan Tan, and bred by Wilma Baron of Gentree Kennel.

Betsy and Jim Wahlberg, Colorado: Cambridge

Betsy and Jim began in English Cockers in 1981, when they bought a little blue roan puppy from Joann Berry's Bangor Kennels. By the time he was two years old, Bangor Cambridge Corker had won his American and Canadian championships, an Award of Merit at the English Cocker Spaniel Club of America Specialty, and his Companion Dog title.

In 1982 Rochan Cambridge Sparkley, a blue roan and tan bitch, joined Cambridge. Shown by Jim to most of her wins, she completed her championship at fifteen months of age and went on to earn a CD degree. Bred to Ch. Reklawholm Rockbeat, she produced Ch. Cambridge Breakdance and Ch. Cambridge Barbary Beat.

In 1984 Ch. Brownhaven Reverie A L'Orange, an orange roan bitch leased from Susie Vallier, was bred to Ch. Stardust Silver Dollar. From that litter of seven puppies four became champions. Both Ch. Cambridge Little Blu Audrey and Ch. Cambridge Ariel Stoutheart, CD, reside with Betsy and Jim. Audrey in turn was bred to Ch. Glenwood's Sierra Echo and whelped five pups in February 1987. Several of these puppies are proving their worth for Cambridge in the show ring.

Also residing at Cambridge is Ch. Lynann's Pacific Pizzazz, a light-blue roan bitch co-owned with Lynda Gall; and Ch. Blue Vu Cambridge Crystalight, bred and co-owned with Lori Capron.

Prudence Walker, British Columbia: Reklawholm

Prudence Walker began breeding English Cockers in the 1930s in England and over the years has developed a worldwide reputation for producing sound dogs with steady, reliable temperaments that can perform in the field, as well as look attractive in the show ring. Her dogs have been instrumental in bloodlines from Finland to New Zealand.

Mrs. Walker emigrated to Canada in the mid-1970s, bringing with her several dogs who were destined to play an important role in

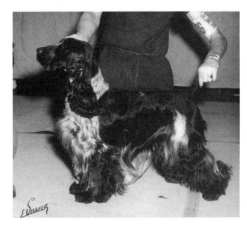

Ch. Kenobo Constellation, blue roan dog (Ch. Dunelm Galaxy ex Ch. Kenobo Moonlight Majic). *Evelyn M. Shafer*

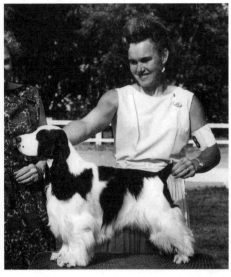

Ch. Reklawholm Paul Jones, black and white dog (Ch. Courtdale Flag Lieutenant ex Reklawholm Tarantella). *Evelyn M. Shafer*

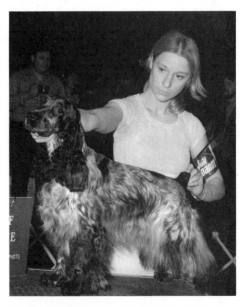

Ch. Bluebell Caryn, blue roan bitch (Ch. Surrey Blue Stone ex Ch. Bluebell Irish Mist). *John L. Ashbey*

the development of the English Cocker in America. Among the most famous was Ch. Reklawholm Paul Jones, who was bred by Mrs. Walker in 1968 and sold to Arthur and Jane Ferguson. He had an excellent show career and produced fourteen champion sons, the most famous being Ch. Applewyn Angus. He was the sire of Reklawholm Poptune, a good producer who was the dam of Am. & Can. Ch. Reklawholm Lyric of Ranzfel, owned by Ann Eldredge of Maidavale Kennels. Another outstanding Reklawholm dog was Firebird, also owned by the Fergusons, who was the sire of more than fifty-eight champions.

Among the current winners and producers from Prudence Walker's kennels is Am. & Can. Ch. Reklawholm Rockbeat, owned by R. and G. Wharton. Rockbeat is the product of a Firebird grandson bred to a Firebird daughter and has nine champions to his credit at this time. Among his outstanding get are Ch. Sweet Apple Ben Davis, Best in Sweepstakes at the 1988 English Cocker Spaniel Club National Specialty; Ch. Jaybriar's Sonnet; and Ch. Reklawholm Royal Blues.

Prudence Walker's success has been built on a simple philosophy: Never buy any animal unless you are fully conversant with the Standard of the breed; never keep any animal that you have to apologize for, it costs no more to feed a good one than a poor one. She also believes a top specimen looks good all over, not in parts. Beware of people who praise its head, front, rear, etc. All parts should measure up to a good whole dog. And finally, never breed from a Cocker that has any exaggeration at all. Always select for dogs that are attractive, powerful, amiable and free of extremes.

Karen M. Ward, California: Happiness Country

Karen has owned English Cockers as pets for twenty-five years but has only been involved in showing them for the past eight years. She is specializing in the orange roan–colored English Cockers. Her foundation bitch, Ch. Dorbert's Joy of Happiness, was bred to BISS Ch. Dickens Tom Wildspark and produced Ch. Happiness' Town Constable and Ch. HCK's Strawberry Shortcake, both orange roans. Ch. Happiness' Town Constable has champion, Group-placing and several major-pointed offspring that are now being shown.

Kathy Wolf, Wisconsin

Kathy Wolf started showing Carachelle Crockett in the spring of 1976. Although he did quite well with Kathy, due to a lack of major points in that area of the country he was sent to California, where he was shown by Ted and Jodelle Burke, the owners of his sire. There he completed his championship with two five-point major wins shortly after his first birthday. As a sire, although limited to a few bitches due to time and space, he produced ten champions.

Two other English Cockers reside with Kathy, Ch. Glenwood's Autumn Brooke and Sleepy Eye Harlequinade.

Cheryl Wright, Virginia

Cheryl is very grateful to Pam Dahl and Carol Lewis, the breeders of Ch. Timmara Doolin' Dalton Cara-Lee, for giving her the opportunity to own this beautiful English Cocker.

Dalton's ring debut resulted in a Best in Sweepstakes win, and he completed his championship on his second birthday. Dalton's other wins include Best of Breed and an English Cocker Spaniel Club of America Award of Merit. In very limited breeding, Dalton has produced champions and major-pointed puppies from each of his litters.

Dalton lives with Cheryl and his two housemates, Carachelle Caprice and Foxfyre Color My World.

Greg and Mary Wysocki, New Jersey: Foxhollow

Greg and Mary purchased their first English Cocker from Maurie and Seymour Prager in 1972. This dog, Ch. On Time Ben's Bluebell Toby, became their first champion.

Their foundation bitch, Ch. Bluebell Caryn, was acquired from Betty Batchelder of Bluebell Kennels. Although bred only a few times, the English Cocker Spaniel Club of America honored her as a top producer in 1981 and 1982. Among her most famous get are Ch. Bluebell Irish Tweed, sired by Ch. Amawalk Cottleston Concorde, and co-bred and owned by Betty Batchelder; and the following dogs sired by Ch. Maidavale Firethorne: Ch. Foxhollow Firecracker; Ch. Penwood Foxhollow I'm Mr. Blu, owned by Lauren and Frank Sorrentino; and Ch. Bluebell Firebrand, owned by Margaret Ritch.

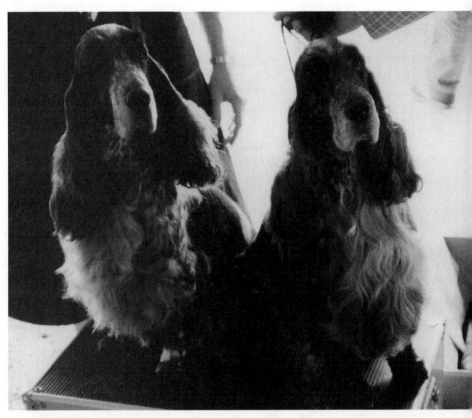

Ch. Kenobo Rabbit of Nadou, age twelve, and Ch. Kenobo Capricorn, age ten—a rare photo of father and son. Between them they sired more than 175 champions, creating a dynasty of quality in the breed that may never be equaled.

12

Selected Pedigrees of Important Sires and Dams

$\mathbf{A}$ PEDIGREE is only important as a symbol of the dog it portrays. Unless one is familiar with the dog represented on the printed page, a pedigree is as meaningless as Egyptian hieroglyphics without the Rosetta stone. It is important, therefore, to try to study by photo and by seeing the dog itself, the animal represented by its pedigree. Many of the dogs included on these pages are no longer with us, but they were so important to the development of the breed in this country that no book would be complete without them.

Among them are the most prominent sires, such as Ch. Kenobo Capricorn, who sired 120 champions, more than any other in the breed. Also included are Ch. Dunelm Galaxy, with 93 champions to his credit, and Ch. Reklawholm Firebird, with 58. Many of the same dogs appear in different pedigrees, because their influence has spread throughout every line in the United States.

Prominent bitches are recognized, too. Ch. Somerset's Saga Antigone, with 21 champions produced, a record for the breed, and Ch. Vari's Fascination, with 14, whose lineage is traced through many families down to the present.

We have also included dogs and bitches who were not among the top producers but who made contributions through their progeny, nonetheless. We include relative newcomers whose produce is likely to influence the breed in years to come.

These pedigrees are by no means a complete compendium of all the English Cockers worthy of recognition, but many of them can be found in the backgrounds of the present generation and so are included here.

Acknowledgment is given to K-9 Bytes, Pasadena, Maryland, for printing out the pedigree information.

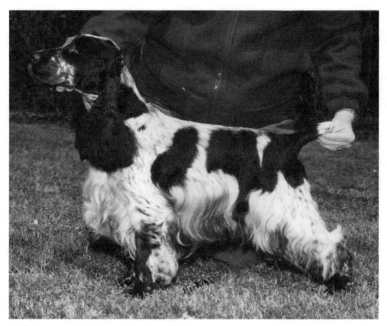

Ch. Kvammes Hollywood, TD (9/26/84).   *Bruce K. Harkins*

CH. KENOBO CAPRICORN
CH. RANZFEL NEWSFLASH, TD
CH. RANZFEL BLUE ROXANNE
CH. CARACHELLE COURT JESTER, WD
CH. CYGNET'S COPPERSTRIKE
CH. CARACHELLE COQUETTE
CH. KENOBO CARITA OF CARACHELLE
AM. & CAN. CH. OLDE SPICE CRUSADER
   (Sire)   CH. REKLAWHOLM PAUL JONES
CH. CARACHELLE CASINO
CH. CARACHELLE COQUETTE
CH. CINDIONE ANDREA CHRISTINE
CH. SOHO INSTANT REPLAY
SOHO REFRAIN
SOHO LYRIC

CH. DUNELM GALAXY
CH. KENOBO CAPRICORN
CH. KENOBO SILVER CHARM
CH. WINGSLADE KVAMMES SPIRIT, TD
CH. DUNELM GALAXY
CH. KENOBO A TOUCH OF MAGIC
CH. KENOBO MOONLIGHT MAJIC
CH. KVAMMES RAZZLE DAZZLE, TD
   (Dam)   REKLAWHOLM HORNPIPE
CH. COPPERALLY MINSTREL OF REKLAWHOLM
COPPERALLY CAMPARI
CH. KVAMME'S ASTRAL, TD
WINGSLADE BLUE SILK N' SAFFRON

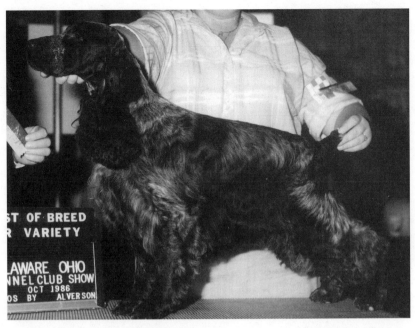

Ch. Daisymead's Dynasty (5/13/84).   *Alverson Photographers, Inc.*

CH. KENOBO CAPRICORN
CH. RANZFEL NEWSFLASH, TD
CH. RANZFEL BLUE ROXANNE
CH. CARACHELLE COURT JESTER, WD
CH. CYGNET'S COPPERSTRIKE
CH. CARACHELLE COQUETTE
CH. KENOBO CARITA OF CARACHELLE
AM. & CAN. CH. OLDE SPICE CRUSADER
(Sire)   CH. REKLAWHOLM PAUL JONES
CH. CARACHELLE CASINO
CH. CARACHELLE COQUETTE
CH. CINDIONE ANDREA CHRISTINE
CH. SOHO INSTANT REPLAY
SOHO REFRAIN
SOHO LYRIC

CH. ASCOT'S DONNY OF SQUIRREL RUN
CH. SURREY BLUE STONE
CH. SURREY BLUE HEN
CH. ROUNDELAY RIVAL
CH. DUNELM GALAXY
CH. DUNELM STARLIGHT
CH. REKLAWHOLM SWINGTIME
CH. DAISYMEAD'S BLUE VELVET
(Dam)   CH. DUNELM PYGMALION
CH. DUNELM GALAXY
CH. DUNELM STARDUST
CH. CANTERBURY'S RAZZLE DAZZLE
CH. KENOBO CONSTELLATION
CH. VARI'S FASCINATION
CH. VARI'S PARTY TRICKS

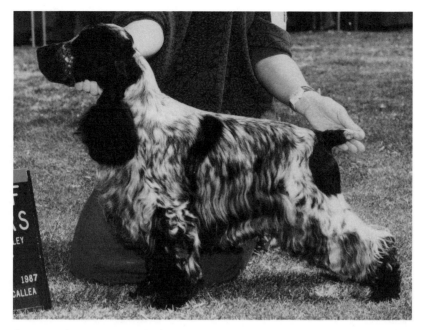

Ch. Lynann's Never Ending Story.   *Callea Photo*

                    CH. KENOBO CAPRICORN
                CH. RANZFEL NEWSFLASH, TD
                    CH. RANZFEL BLUE ROXANNE
        CH. CARACHELLE COURT JESTER, WD
                    CH. CYGNET'S COPPERSTRIKE
                CH. CARACHELLE COQUETTE
                    CH. KENOBO CARITA OF CARACHELLE
AM. & CAN. CH. OLDE SPICE CRUSADER
     (Sire)   CH. REKLAWHOLM PAUL JONES
                CH. CARACHELLE CASINO
                    CH. CARACHELLE COQUETTE
        CH. CINDIONE ANDREA CHRISTINE
                    CH. SOHO INSTANT REPLAY
                SOHO REFRAIN
                    SOHO LYRIC

                    CH. KENOBO CAPRICORN
                ABERGLEN FRONT RUNNER
                    CH. WOODLEA DICROFT PENNYROYAL
        CH. GLENWOOD SIERRA ECHO
                    CH. CARACHELLE COPPER LION
                CH. WYNCASTLE SILVER STARDUST
                    CH. GRAECROFT LEGEND OF WYN-STAR
CH. LYNANN'S PRECIOUS IMAGE
     (Dam)   CH. KENOBO CAPRICORN
            CH. GRAECROFT TARUS OF WYNCASTLE
                    CH. GRAECROFT FEATHER DUSTER
        CH. WYNCASTLE CINDERELLA
                WYNCASTLE CANDILAND

                                                                211

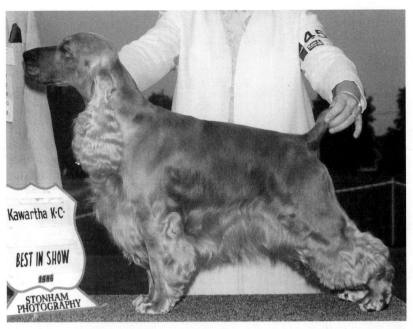

Am. & Can. Ch. Hobbithill Ashwood Hi Class (4/24/84). *Stonham Photography*

CH. JANEACRE NIGHT SKIPPER OF HELENWOOD
LOCHRANZA NIGHT TO REMEMBER
ENG. CH. LOCHRANZA BITTERSWEET
CH. LOCHRANZA MAN OF FASHION
ENG. CH. LOCHRANZA NEWSPRINT
LOCHRANZA DOLLY POSH
PAINTED DOLL OF LOCHRANZA
CH. HUBBESTAD KERMIT
   (Sire)   ENG. CH. BRONZE KNIGHT OF BROOMLEAF
ENG. CH. LOCHRANZA FARMER'S BOY
LOCHRANZA DAIRYMAID
NOR. CH. HUBBESTAD KELDA
NOR. CH. HUBBESTAD JONATHAN
NOR. CH. HUBBESTAD KAREENA
SCAND. CH. HUBBESTAD KATRINKA

CORNBOW MANFRED
SUNGLINT OF SORBROOK
QUETTADENE BERNADETTE
AM. & CAN. CH. SORBROOK DANDYLION
BUTTER PRINT OF BROOMLEAF
BUTTER KIST OF SORBROOK
WISTFUL LASS OF SORBROOK
CH. GAYBROOK AMBER OF HOBBITHILL
   (Dam)   ENG. CH. LOCHRANZA HIGHTREES RED ADMIRAL
CAN. CH. LOCHRANZA KAVORA GAY HUSSAR
KAVORA SUSAN OF SANDOVER
CAN. CH. RANZFEL SINCERELY AMBER
ENG. CH. LOCHRANZA HIGHTREES RED ADMIRAL
CAN. CH. LOCHRANZA DANCING MISTRESS
LOCHRANZA DANCING LESSON

212

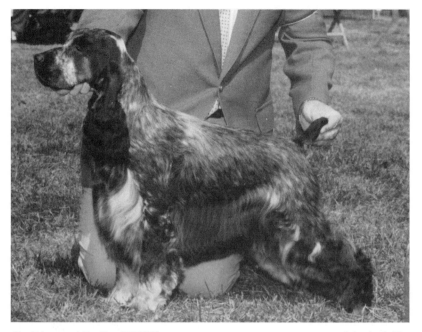

Ch. Edgewood Fan-Tan (5/22/83).   *John L. Ashbey*

```
                    CH. COLINWOOD BLAZE AWAY
          CH. DUNELM PYGMALION
                    COLINWOOD WOODROYD CAROUSEL
    CH. DUNELM GALAXY
                    CH. GLENGLADDON LUCKY STAR
          CH. DUNELM STARDUST
                    DUNELM MERRY-GO-ROUND
CH. KENOBO CAPRICORN
    (Sire)          CH. DUNELM GALAXY
          CH. KENOBO OLIVER LUV
                    CH. KENOBO MOONLIGHT MAJIC
    CH. KENOBO SILVER CHARM
                    CH. BROOKHAVEN BEAU BRUMMEL
          CH. KENOBO CHARM BRACELET
                    COLINWOOD SILVER BANGLE


                    CH. DUNELM PYGMALION
          CH. DUNELM GALAXY
                    CH. DUNELM STARDUST
    CH. KENOBO CAPRICORN
                    CH. KENOBO OLIVER LUV
          CH. KENOBO SILVER CHARM
                    CH. KENOBO CHARM BRACELET
CH. GRAECROFT CALLIOPE
    (Dam)           CH. DUNELM GALAXY
          CH. DUNELM GALLIARD
                    CH. REKLAWHOLM SWINGTIME
    CH. JUNEBUG'S BLUE PIXY
                    CH. ON TIME DORRIE'S LARRY
          JUNEBUG'S COTTON CANDY
                    ON TIME CASSANDRA'S BERYL
```

213

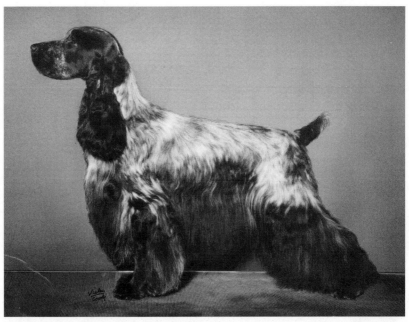

Ch. Wyncastle Lookin At You Kid (4/22/82). *Vicky Cook*

CH. DUNELM PYGMALION
CH. DUNELM GALAXY
CH. DUNELM STARDUST
CH. KENOBO CAPRICORN
CH. KENOBO OLIVER LUV
CH. KENOBO SILVER CHARM
CH. KENOBO CHARM BRACELET
CH. WYNCASTLES PLAY IT AGAIN SAM
(Sire)   CH. GRAECROFT TARUS OF WYNCASTLE
CH. CARACHELLE COPPER LION
CH. KENOBO JOYOUS NOELLE
CH. WYNCASTLES SILVER STARDUST
CH. KENOBO CAPRICORN
CH. GRAECROFT LEGEND OF WYN-STAR
CH. JUNEBUG'S BLUE PIXY

CH. KENOBO CAPRICORN
CH. GRAECROFT TARUS OF WYNCASTLE
CH. GRAECROFT FEATHER DUSTER
CH. CARACHELLE COPPER LION
CH. DUNELM SMOKE SIGNAL OF WENLOE
CH. KENOBO JOYOUS NOELLE
CH. KENOBO STAR STRUCK SHADOW
WYNCASTLES JENNY CHURCHILL
(Dam)   CH. DUNELM GALAXY
CH. KENOBO CAPRICORN
CH. KENOBO SILVER CHARM
CH. GRAECROFT LEGEND OF WYN-STAR
CH. DUNELM GALLIARD
CH. JUNEBUG'S BLUE PIXY
JUNEBUG'S COTTON CANDY

214

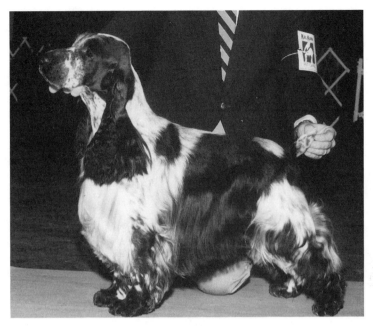

Am. & Can. Ch. Amawalk's Perrocay Qeqertag (7/20/81).   *John L. Ashbey*

```
                    CH. DUNELM PYGMALION
            CH. DUNELM GALAXY
                    CH. DUNELM STARDUST
        CH. KENOBO CAPRICORN
                    CH. KENOBO OLIVER LUV
            CH. KENOBO SILVER CHARM
                    CH. KENOBO CHARM BRACELET
    CH. KENOBO CONFETTI
        (Sire)      CH. DUNELM PYGMALION
            CH. DUNELM GALAXY
                    CH. DUNELM STARDUST
        CH. KENOBO HAPPINESS IS
                    CH. SILVER LARIOT OF STRATHPINE
            CH. KENOBO MOONLIGHT MAJIC
                    CH. CYGNET'S RASPBERRY


                    COURTDALE COLINWOOD SEAHAWK
            ENG. CH. COURTDALE FLAG LIEUTENANT
                    COURTDALE KINKELLBRIDGE GINA
        CH. REKLAWHOLM FIREBIRD
                    REKLAWHOLM SUCU-SUCU
            REKLAWHOLM BLUE RHAPSODY
                    REKLAWHOLM TARANTELLA
    CH. AMAWALK'S KATRINA
        (Dam)       CH. DUNELM GALAXY
            CH. KENOBO CONSTELLATION
                    CH. KENOBO MOONLIGHT MAJIC
        CH. AMAWALK'S LUCKY CHARM
                    CH. COURTDALE BUCCANEER
            ANCRAM'S MUFFIN OF AMAWALK
                    TWILIGHT OF HEARTS
```

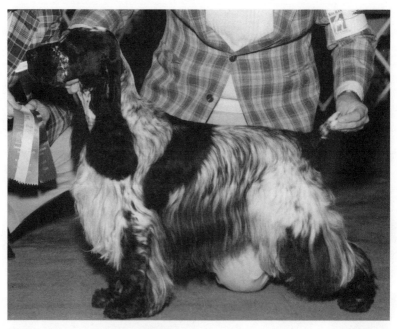

Ch. Reklawholm Rockbeat (10/20/80). *Cott/Francis*

                    COURTDALE COLINWOOD SEAHAWK
            ENG. CH. COURTDALE FLAG LIEUTENANT
                    COURTDALE KINKELLBRIDGE GINA
      CH. REKLAWHOLM FIREBIRD
                    REKLAWHOLM SUCU-SUCU
            REKLAWHOLM BLUE RHAPSODY
                    REKLAWHOLM TARANTELLA
DUNELM DISCO OF REKLAWHOLM
      (Sire)   LEABANK LEVITY
            CH. REKLAWHOLM LYRIC OF RANZFEL
                    REKLAWHOLM POPTUNE
      DUNELM BLOSSON
                    CH. KENOBO CONSTELLATION
            CH. DUNELM MADRIGAL
                    CH. DUNELM STARLIGHT

                    CH. DUNELM GALAXY
            CH. KENOBO CAPRICORN
                    CH. KENOBO SILVER CHARM
      AM. & CAN. CH. RANZFEL NEWSFLASH, TD
                    AM. & CAN. CH. CRAIGLEITH MAGIC FLUTE
            AM. & CAN. CH. RANZFEL BLUE ROXANNE
                    CAN. CH. RANZFEL MEGAN BLUE
CAN. CH. REKLAWHOLM INTERMEZZO
      (Dam)   REKLAWHOLM HORNPIPE
            AM. & CAN. CH. COPPERALLY MINSTRAL OF REK
                    COPPERALLY CAMPARI
      AM. & CAN. CH. REKLAWHOLM REVERIE
                    SCOLY'S STARDUSTER
            AM. & CAN. CH. REKLAWHOLM MIDNIGHT BLUES
                    REKLAWHOLM POPTUNE

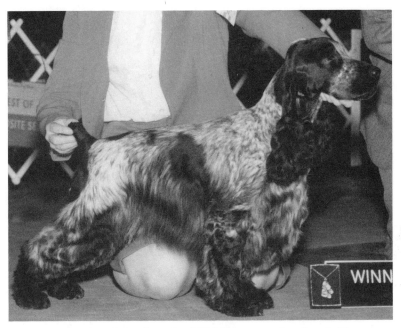

Am. & Can. Ch. Olde Spice Crusader (9/29/80). *Don Petrulis Photography*

CH. DUNELM GALAXY
CH. KENOBO CAPRICORN
CH. KENOBO SILVER CHARM
AM. & CAN. CH. RANZFEL NEWSFLASH, TD
AM. & CAN. CH. CRAIGLEITH MAGIC FLUTE
AM. & CAN. CH. RANZFEL BLUE ROXANNE
CAN. CH. RANZFEL MEGAN BLUE
CH. CARACHELLE COURT JESTER, WD
(Sire) CH. DUNELM PYGMALION
CH. CYGNET'S COPPERSTRIKE
CH. DUNELM DARK STAR
CH. CARACHELLE COQUETTE
CH. KENOBO RABBIT OF NADOU
CH. KENOBO CARITA OF CARACHELLE
CH. KENOBO SILVER CHARM

COURTDALE FLAG LIEUTENANT
CH. REKLAWHOLM PAUL JONES
REKLAWHOLM TARANTELLA
CH. CARACHELLE CASINO
CH. CYGNET'S COPPERSTRIKE
CH. CARACHELLE COQUETTE
CH. KENOBO CARITA OF CARACHELLE
CH. CINDIONE ANDREA CHRISTINE
(Dam) CH. SOHO COUNTERPOINT
CH. SOHO INSTANT REPLAY
CH. SOHO FORTUNE COOKIE
SOHO REFRAIN
CH. SOHO MARKSMAN OF WYNCREST
SOHO LYRIC
SOHO STARMIST

217

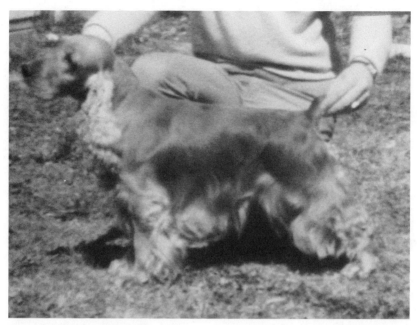

Ch. Hubbestad Kermit (7/29/80).

```
                          SUNGLINT OF SORBROOK
              CH. JANEACRE NIGHT SKIPPER OF HELENWOOD
                     JANEACRE MAID MARION OF LOCHNELL
        LOCHRANZA NIGHT TO REMEMBER
                     ENG. CH. LOCHRANZA QUETTADANE MARKSMAN
              ENG. CH. LOCHRANZA BITTERSWEET
                     LOCHRANZA MONKSPRING MARIGOLD
CH. LOCHRANZA MAN OF FASHION
     (Sire)          BUTTER PRINT OF BROOMLEAD
              ENG. CH. LOCHRANZA NEWSPRINT
                     ENG. CH. LOCHRANZA BITTERSWEET
        LOCHRANZA DOLLY POSH
                     LOCHRANZA BARSAC FARRIER
              PAINTED DOLL OF LOCHRANZA
                     LOCHRANZA TAN SLIPPERS



                          ENG. CH. SCOTSWOOD WARLORD
              ENG. CH. BRONZE KNIGHT OF BROOMLEAF
                     BLACKFROST OF BROOMLEAF
        ENG. CH. LOCHRANZA FARMER'S BOY
                     BUTTER PRINT OF BROOMLEAF
              LOCHRANZA DAIRYMAID
                     ENG. CH. LOCHRANZA BITTERSWEET
NOR. CH. HUBBESTAD KELDA
     (Dam)           INT. CH. LOCHDENE KESTILA
              NOR. CH. HUBBESTAD JONATHAN
                     INT. CH. MOORCLIFFE MODEL RED
        NOR. CH. HUBBESTAD KAREENA
                     NOR. & SWED. CH. ORLIDERS DANCING STAR
              SCAND. CH. HUBBESTAD KATRINKA
                     MORWENS NIGGER GIRL OF WARE
```

218

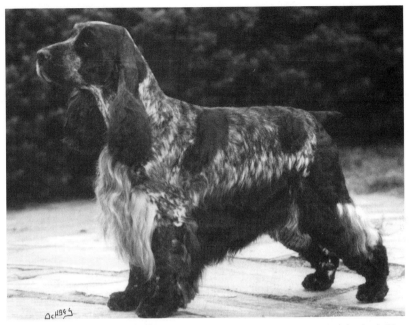

Ch. Maidavale Firethorne (5/3/77). *John L. Ashbey*

ENG. CH. COLINWOOD SILVER LARIOT
COURTDALE COLINWOOD SEAHAWK
ORBURN SEA FOAM
ENG. CH. COURTDALE FLAG LIEUTENANT
WELLS FARGO OF WEIRDENE
COURTDALE KINKELLBRIDGE GINA
KINKELLBRIDGE TOSKA
CH. REKLAWHOLM FIREBIRD
(Sire)   GOLDENFIELDS MINSTREL BOY
REKLAWHOLM SUCU-SUCU
REKLAWHOLM FLAMENCO
REKLAWHOLM BLUE RHAPSODY
CAN. CH. CRAIGLEITH VAGABOND KING
REKLAWHOLM TARANTELLA
REKLAWHOLM PETRONELLA

CH. COLINWOOD BLAZE AWAY
CH. DUNELM PYGMALION
COLINWOOD WOODROYD CAROUSEL
CH. DUNELM GALAXY
CH. GLENGLADDON LUCKY STAR
CH. DUNELM STARDUST
DUNELM MERRY-GO-ROUND
CH. MAIDAVALE TIFFIN
(Dam)   CH. SQUIRREL RUN THORN
CH. ASCOT'S DONNY OF SQUIRREL RUN
PAGE'S KANDY KISS
CH. SURREY BLUE JEAN
CH. DUNELM GALAXY
CH. SURREY BLUE HEN
DUNELM SURREY GAMBIT

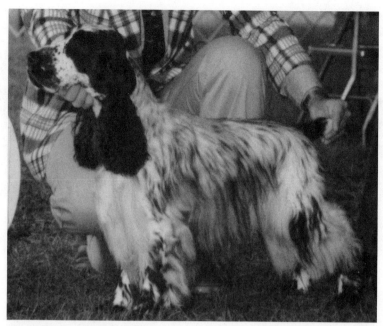

Ch. Applewyn Angus (2/12/75). *Dick and Diana Alverson*

```
                    ENG. CH. COLINWOOD SILVER LARIOT
              COURTDALE COLINWOOD SEAHAWK
                    ORBURN SEA FOAM
           ENG. CH. COURTDALE FLAG LIEUTENANT
                    WELLS FARGO OF WEIRDENE
              COURTDALE KINKELLBRIDGE GINA
                    KINKELLBRIDGE TOSKA
     CH. REKLAWHOLM PAUL JONES
        (Sire)    CAN. CH. CRAIGLEITH VAGABOND KING
              REKLAWHOLM TARANTELLA
                    REKLAWHOLM PETRONELLA



                    COURTDALE COLINWOOD SEAHAWK
              ENG. CH. COURTDALE FLAG LIEUTENANT
                    COURTDALE KINKELLBRIDGE GINA
           THE MATAROA OF MERRYBRAY
                    COURTDALE COLINWOOD SEAHAWK
              MERRYBRAY HONEYSUCKLE
                    MERRYBRAY MELROSE
     CH. RANDLINE BLUE MIST OF MERRYBRAY
        (Dam)          ENG. CH. LUCKLENA BLUE MUSIC
              LUCKLENA ROYDWOOD RICH RELATION
                    ROYDWOOD REMARKABLE
           RANDLINE BLUE DAPHNE
                    RANDLINE DOMINATOR
              RANDLINE DONNA
                    RANDLINE WINONA
```

220

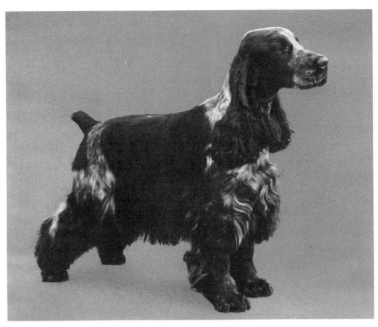

Am. & Can. Ch. Ranzfel Newsflash, TD (11/11/75).

```
                    CH. COLINWOOD BLAZE AWAY
          CH. DUNELM PYGMALION
                    COLINWOOD WOODROYD CAROUSEL
    CH. DUNELM GALAXY
                    CH. GLENGLADDON LUCKY STAR
          CH. DUNELM STARDUST
                    DUNELM MERRY-GO-ROUND
CH. KENOBO CAPRICORN
     (Sire)         CH. DUNELM GALAXY
          CH. KENOBO OLIVER LUV
                    CH. KENOBO MOONLIGHT MAJIC
    CH. KENOBO SILVER CHARM
                    CH. BROOKHAVEN BEAU BRUMMEL
          CH. KENOBO CHARM BRACELET
                    COLINWOOD SILVER BANGLE


                    CRAGLEITH MASQUERADE
          CRAIGLEITH TALK OF THE TOWN
                    ENG. CH. CRAIGLEITH SWEET CHARITY
    AM. & CAN. CH. CRAIGLEITH MAGIC FLUTE
                    GLENCORA MAYHILL MALLORY
          TUDOR GOLD FLUTE OBLIGATO
                    TUDOR GOLD CRAIGLEITH FLIORELLO
AM. & CAN. CH. RANZFEL BLUE ROXANNE
     (Dam)          ENG. CH. COURTDALE FLAG LIEUTENANT
          AM. & CAN. CH. COLINWOOD COASTGUARD
                    COLINWOOD PERCHANCE
    CAN. CH. RANZFEL MEGAN BLUE
                    ENG. CH. WEIRDANE QUESTING STRATHSPEY
          CAN. CH. WILLOWBANK CALLIE OF RANZFEL
                    CAN. CH. COCHISE CARIOCA
```

221

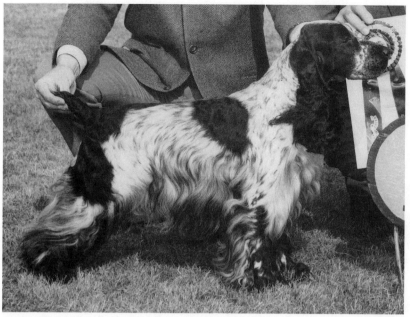

Ch. Dunelm Galaxy (10/5/64). *Evelyn M. Shafer*

```
                    ENG. CH. BLACKMOOR BRAND
             COLINWOOD FIREBRAND
                    COLINWOOD CIGARETTE
       CH. COLINWOOD BLAZE AWAY
                    COLINWOOD JESTER OF GLENBOGIE
             TRUSLER'S TRACERY
                    TRIXIE OF TRUSLERS
CH. DUNELM PYGMALION
      (Sire)          BLACKMOOR BRAND
             BRIARCLIFFE BENET
                    LOVERSALL EXQUISITE
       COLINWOOD WOODROYD CAROUSEL
                    ENG. CH. COLINWOOD COWBOY
             WOODROYD BALLERINA
                    BLUE JENNY OF GLOURIE


                    ENG. CH. DOMINO OF IDE
             VALSTAR LUCKLENA MINSTREL
                    LUCKLENA MELODIOUS MAID
       CH. GLENGLADDON LUCKY STAR
                    AM. & CAN. CH. COLINWOOD JOKER
             GLENGLADDON BLUE DIANA
                    COLINWOOD FESTOON
CH. DUNELM STARDUST
      (Dam)          CH. ELBLAC'S BUGLE OF HASTERN
             CH. JOYANNE'S DANIEL OF DUNELM
                    CH. GRAYERLIN'S ANONYMOUS
       DUNELM MERRY-GO-ROUND
                    BRIARCLIFFE BENET
             COLINWOOD WOODROYD CAROUSEL
                    WOODROYD BALLERINA
```

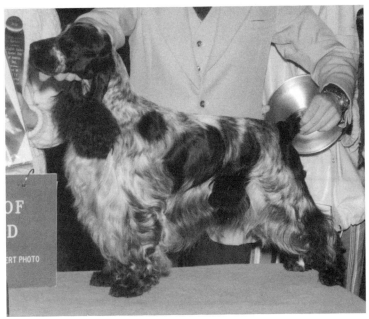

Ch. Aberschan's Reginald (6/22/74).   *Gilbert Photo*

                CH. COLINWOOD BLAZE AWAY
            CH. DUNELM PYGMALION
                COLINWOOD WOODROYD CAROUSEL
        CH. DUNELM GALAXY
                CH. GLENGLADDON LUCKY STAR
            CH. DUNELM STARDUST
                DUNELM MERRY-GO-ROUND
    CH. KENOBO CAPRICORN
        (Sire)   CH. DUNELM GALAXY
            CH. KENOBO OLIVER LUV
                CH. KENOBO MOONLIGHT MAJIC
        CH. KENOBO SILVER CHARM
                CH. BROOKHAVEN BEAU BRUMMEL
            CH. KENOBO CHARM BRACELET
                COLINWOOD SILVER BANGLE

                CH. COLINWOOD BLAZE AWAY
            CH. DUNELM PYGMALION
                COLINWOOD WOODROYD CAROUSEL
        CH. DUNELM GALAXY
                CH. GLENGLADDON LUCKY STAR
            CH. DUNELM STARDUST
                DUNELM MERRY-GO-ROUND
    CH. ABERSCHAN TUPPENCE OF YORK
        (Dam)   ANCRAM'S PIPPIN
        ANCRAM'S JESSICA
                CH. SILVER LARIOT OF STRATHPINE
            ANCRAM'S AMANDA
                RICMOUR CRYSTAL DAWN

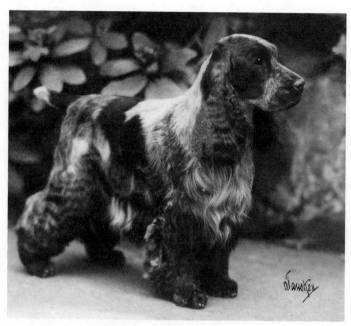

Ch. Kenobo Capricorn (1/1/72). *Tausky*

CH. COLINWOOD BLAZE AWAY
CH. DUNELM PYGMALION
COLINWOOD WOODROYD CAROUSEL
CH. DUNELM GALAXY
CH. GLENGLADDON LUCKY STAR
CH. DUNELM STARDUST
DUNELM MERRY-GO-ROUND
CH. KENOBO RABBIT OF NADOU
(Sire)   CH. COLINWOOD CHEYENNE
CH. DUNELM HICKORY
CH. DUNELM CHEROKEE ROSE
CH. CYGNET'S RASPBERRY, CD
CH. QUARTO L. ALERT'S SON
SOHO BATIK
CH. ON TIME'S OWN ANNIE

CH. DUNELM PYGMALION
CH. DUNELM GALAXY
CH. DUNELM STARDUST
CH. KENOBO OLIVER LUV
CH. SILVER LARIOT OF STRATHPINE
CH. KENOBO MOONLIGHT MAJIC
CH. CYGNET'S RASPBERRY, CD
CH. KENOBO SILVER CHARM
(Dam)   CH. SILVER LARIOT OF STRATHPINE
CH. BROOKHAVEN BEAU BRUMMEL
VICKI OF KEN-LYN
CH. KENOBO CHARM BRACELET
COLINWOOD WRANGLER
COLINWOOD SILVER BANGLE
COLINWOOD SILVER CIRCLET

224

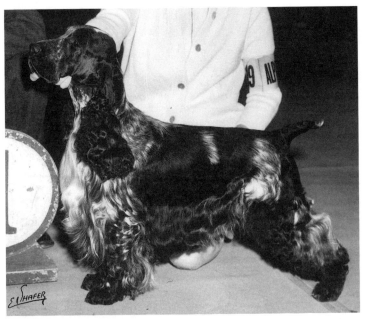

Ch. Kenobo Rabbit of Nadou (2/28/69).   *Evelyn M. Shafer*

```
                        COLINWOOD FIREBRAND
                  CH. COLINWOOD BLAZE AWAY
                        TRUSLER'S TRACERY
            CH. DUNELM PYGMALION
                        BRIARCLIFFE BENET
                  COLINWOOD WOODROYD CAROUSEL
                        WOODROYD BALLERINA
      CH. DUNELM GALAXY
            (Sire)       VALSTAR LUCKLENA MINSTREL
                  CH. GLENGLADDON LUCKY STAR
                        GLENGLADDON BLUE DIANA
            CH. DUNELM STARDUST
                        CH. JOYANNE'S DANIEL OF DUNELM
                  DUNELM MERRY-GO-ROUND
                        COLINWOOD WOODROYD CAROUSEL


                        ENG. CH. COLINWOOD SILVER LARIOT
                  CH. COLINWOOD CHEYENNE
                        CRAIGLEITH GEISHA GIRL
            CH. DUNELM HICKORY
                        CH. JOYANNE'S DANIEL OF DUNELM
                  CH. DUNELM CHEROKEE ROSE
                        CH. DUNELM DAPHNE
      CH. CYGNET'S RASPBERRY, CD
            (Dam)       CH. SKY RIDGE ALERT
                  CH. QUARTO L. ALERT'S SON
                        STEVELYN SOLANGE
            SOHO BATIK
                        CH. ON TIME WILLIE II
                  CH. ON TIME'S OWN ANNIE
                        CH. ON TIME DEBORAH
```

225

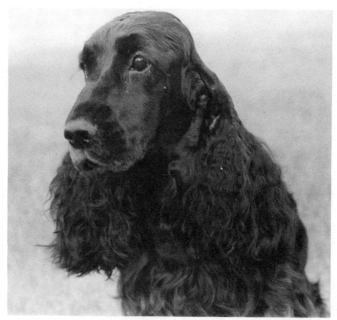

Am. & Can. Ch. Merryborne Minstrel, WDX (9/28/72). © *Linda Wasko, 1981*

ENG. CH. LOCHRANZA HIGHTREES RED ADMIRAL
   ENG. CH. LOCHRANZA STROLLAWAY
      LOCHRANZA DANCING LESSON
  BRAZ. CH. MERRYBORNE STROLLALONG
      ENG. CH. COLINWOOD JACKDAW OF LOCHNELL
     MERRYBORNE MICHELE
      MERRYBORNE COLINWOOD HILLFLOWER
MERRYBORNE MANTAN
  (Sire)   ENG. CH. LOCHRANZA QUETTADENE MARKSMAN
     AM. & CAN. CH. MERRYBORNE BIG SHOT
      LOCHRANZA HONEYGLOW
   TAKE A CHANCE OF ANDANA
      FIGARO OF ANDANA
     CLAUSENTUM GOLDEN TANSY
      CLAUSENTUM GOLDEN CHANCE

ENG. CH. LOCHRANZA HIGHTREES RED ADMIRAL
   ENG. CH. LOCHRANZA DARNCLEVER
      LOCHRANZA DANCING LESSON
  CH. MERRYBORNE MASTERPIECE
      ENG. CH. LOCHRANZA MERRYLEAF EIGAR
     MERRYBORNE MARTINE
      LOCHRANZA HONEYGLOW
MERRYBORNE MAXINE
  (Dam)   ENG. CH. VALJOKER OF MISBOURNE
     BRAZ. CH. COLINWOOD BLACK EAGLE
      COLINWOOD MOORHEN
   MERRYBORNE COLINWOOD HILLFLOWER
      COLINWOOD RICLAR SCARLET PIMPERNEL
     COLINWOOD SUNSET
      COLINWOOD RED ROSE

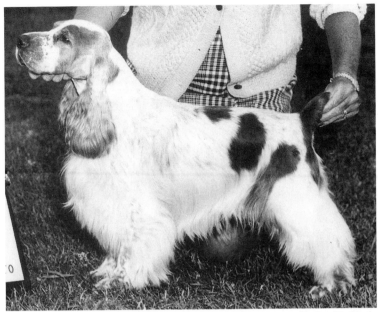

Ch. Reklawholm Firebird (7/1/70). *Evelyn M. Shafer*

JOYWYN'S BLUE FLASH
ENG. CH. COLINWOOD SILVER LARIOT
TRUSLERS MISTY MORN
COURTDALE COLINWOOD SEAHAWK
COLINWOOD DARNMILL DANDY TIM
ORBURN SEA FOAM
ORBURN FIREFLY
ENG. CH. COURTDALE FLAG LIEUTENANT
(Sire)   WEIRDENE BARNSCAR FISHER
WELLS FARGO OF WEIRDENE
WEIRDENE TRECH ZENDA
COURTDALE KINKELLBRIDGE GINA
KINKELLBRIDGE BLUEBOTTLE
KINKELLBRIDGE TOSKA
KINKELLBRIDGE SUNFLOWER

ENG. CH. JOYWYN'S BLUE BOY OF WARE
GOLDENFIELDS MINSTREL BOY
ENG. CH. GOLDENFIELDS MERRY MAIDEN
REKLAWHOLM SUCU-SUCU
REKLAWHOLM FLAMENCO
REKLAWHOLM BLUE RHAPSODY
(Dam)   GOLDENFIELD'S MINSTREL BOY
CRAIGLEITH VAGABOND KING
CRAIGLEITH HEATHERMAID
REKLAWHOLM TARANTELLA
REKLAWHOLM PETRONELLA

227

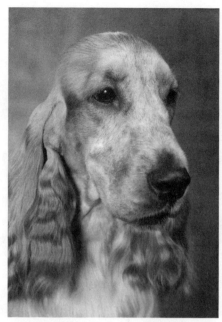
Ch. Brownhaven Reverie A L'Orange.

COURTDALE COLINWOOD SEAHAWK
ENG. CH. COURTDALE FLAG LIEUTENANT
COURTDALE KINKELLBRIDGE GINA
CH. REKLAWHOLM FIREBIRD
REKLAWHOLM SUCU-SUCU
REKLAWHOLM BLUE RHAPSODY
REKLAWHOLM TARANTELLA
CH. MAIDAVALE FIRETHORNE
(Sire)   CH. DUNELM PYGMALION
CH. DUNELM GALAXY
CH. DUNELM STARDUST
CH. MAIDAVALE TIFFIN
CH. ASCOT'S DONNY OF SQUIRREL RUN
CH. SURREY BLUE JEAN
CH. SURREY BLUE HEN

CH. DUNELM GALAXY
CH. KENOBO CAPRICORN
CH. KENOBO SILVER CHARM
CH. GRAECROFT TARUS OF WYNCASTLE
CH. KENOBO RABBIT OF NADOU
CH. GRAECROFT FEATHER DUSTER
CH. JUNEBUG'S BLUE PIXY
CH. CONNEMARA SWEET CHARITY BRWN
(Dam)   WAYMASTER OF WEIRDENE
CH. SHENANDOAH SEAFARER
SHENANDOAH SUNKIST
CH. CONNEMARA SWEET SURRENDER
CH. KENOBO RABBIT OF NADOU
CH. GRAECROFT CONNEMARA SUNSHINE
CH. JUNEBUG'S BLUE PIXY

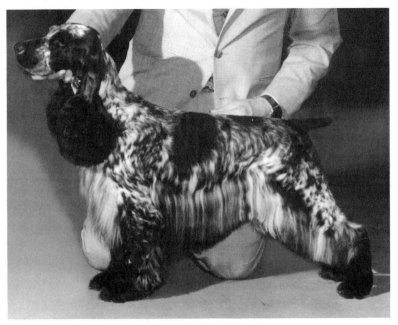

Ch. Sweet Apple Granny Smith (12/1/81).

```
                         CH. ALLEGRA WINDSTORM, TD
                 CH. APPLEWYN ADJUTANT, CD
                         CH. RANDLINE BLUE MIST OF MERRYBRAE
         CH. APPLEWYN ARGYLE
                         CH. RANDLINE GAME DEAL
                 CH. BIRCHWYN BONUS
                         BIRCHWYN BLUE STAR II
CH. PRIDE ACRES LORD GRADY BRICE
      (Sire)            THE MATAROA OF MERRYBRAY
                 CH. RANDLINE GAME DEAL
                         RANDLINE BLUE DAPHNE
         CH. PRIDE ACRES LADY BEVIN GALEN
                         CH. ALLEGRA WINDSTORM, TD
                 CH. BIRCHWYN BRIDGID OF KILDARE
                         BIRCHWYN BLUE STAR II


                         CH. DUNELM PYGMALION
                 CH. DUNELM GALAXY
                         CH. DUNELM STARDUST
         CH. KENOBO CAPRICORN
                         CH. KENOBO OLIVER LUV
                 CH. KENOBO SILVER CHARM
                         CH. KENOBO CHARM BRACELET
CH. ASHGROVE ABIGAIL BLUE
      (Dam)             CH. ASCOT'S DONNY OF SQUIRREL RUN
                 CH. SURREY BLUE STONE
                         CH. SURREY BLUE HEN
         CH. ASHGROVE AMOURETTE
                         CH. BIRCHWYN BOO TOO OF MARMONTS
                 CH. PEACHES N CREAM OF ASHGROVE
                         CH. HARWELL MANOR TASTY TRIFLE, CD
```

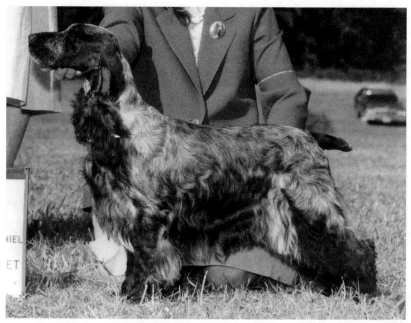

Ch. Parade Pegeen, CDX (3/27/79).   *Janet Ashbey*

```
                         CH. DUNELM PYGMALION
                    CH. DUNELM GALAXY
                         CH. DUNELM STARDUST
               CH. KENOBO RABBIT OF NADOU
                         CH. DUNELM HICKORY
                    CH. CYGNET'S RASPBERRY, CD
                         SOHO BATIK
          CH. PRIDE ACRES LORD EGAN BRAEMAR
               (Sire)        CH. DUNELM DICTATOR
                    CH. ALLEGRA WINDSTORM, TD
                         CH. SHIKAR WYN'S SCILLA, CDX, TD
               CH. BIRCHWYN BRAEMAR
                         THE MATAROA OF MERRYBRAY
                    CH. RANDLINE BLUE MIST OF MERRYBRAE
                         RANDLINE BLUE DAPHNE


                         CH. DUNELM PYGMALION
                    CH. DUNELM GALAXY
                         CH. DUNELM STARDUST
               CH. CANTERBURY'S GENTRY
                         CH. KENOBO CONSTELLATION
                    CH. VARI'S FASCINATION
                         CH. VARI'S PARTY TRICKS
          CH. PARADE DREAMBOAT ANNIE
               (Dam)        CH. ASCOT'S DONNY OF SQUIRREL RUN
                    CH. SURREY BLUE STONE
                         CH. SURREY BLUE HEN
               CH. A TRACE OF WITCH BEWARE
                         CH. LONG VIEW ACRES THREE SPOT
                    CH. SURREY BLUE WITCH
                         DUNELM SURREY GAMBIT
```

230

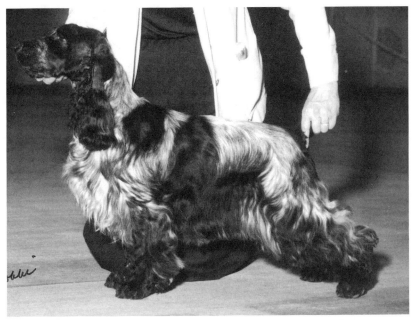

Ch. Tin-Star's My Lil' Chickadee (11/26/78).   *Carl Lindemaier*

ENG. CH. COLINWOOD SILVER LARIOT
COURTDALE COLINWOOD SEAHAWK
ORBURN SEA FOAM
ENG. CH. COURTDALE FLAG LIEUTENANT
WELLS FARGO OF WEIRDENE
COURTDALE KINKELLBRIDGE GINA
KINKELLBRIDGE TOSKA
CH. REKLAWHOLM FIREBIRD
    (Sire)   GOLDENFIELDS MINSTREL BOY
REKLAWHOLM SUCU-SUCU
REKLAWHOLM FLAMENCO
REKLAWHOLM BLUE RHAPSODY
CAN. CH. CRAIGLEITH VAGABOND KING
REKLAWHOLM TARANTELLA
REKLAWHOLM PETRONELLA

CH. SQUIRREL RUN THORN
CH. ASCOT'S DONNY OF SQUIRREL RUN
PAGE'S KANDY KISS
CH. SURREY BLUE STONE
CH. DUNELM GALAXY
CH. SURREY BLUE HEN
DUNELM SURREY GAMBIT
CH. PAGANHILL INSPIRATION, CD, TD
    (Dam)   JOYWYN'S BLUE FLASH
CH. LOCHNELL BLUE FLASH OF ULWELL
TORTAL OF ULWELL
CH. PAGAN HILL FLOWER CHILD, UDT
CH. MAPLE LAWN WINNING TICKET
CH. SOHO SPECULATION
CH. SOHO BEGUILING

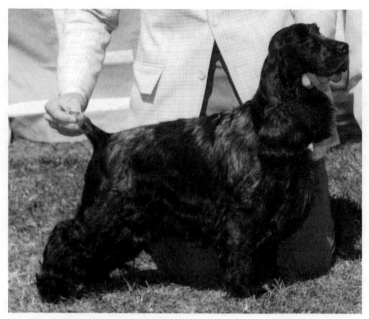

Ch. Graecroft Calliope (11/7/74).   *Michael Enterprises*

                    CH. COLINWOOD BLAZE AWAY
            CH. DUNELM PYGMALION
                    COLINWOOD WOODROYD CAROUSEL
        CH. DUNELM GALAXY
                    CH. GLENGLADDON LUCKY STAR
            CH. DUNELM STARDUST
                    DUNELM MERRY-GO-ROUND
    CH. KENOBO CAPRICORN
        (Sire)   CH. DUNELM GALAXY
            CH. KENOBO OLIVER LUV
                    CH. KENOBO MOONLIGHT MAJIC
        CH. KENOBO SILVER CHARM
                    CH. BROOKHAVEN BEAU BRUMMEL
            CH. KENOBO CHARM BRACELET
                    COLINWOOD SILVER BANGLE

                    CH. DUNELM PYGMALION
            CH. DUNELM GALAXY
                    CH. DUNELM STARDUST
        CH. DUNELM GALLIARD
                    REKLAWHOLM SUCU-SUCU
            CH. REKLAWHOLM SWINGTIME
                    REKLAWHOLM TARANTELLA
    CH. JUNEBUG'S BLUE PIXY
        (Dam)   CH. ON TIME ANNETTE'S LESLIE
            CH. ON TIME DORRIE'S LARRY
                    CH. ON TIME DORRIE
        JUNEBUG'S COTTON CANDY
                    CH. ON TIME ANNETTE'S BILL
            ON TIME CASSANDRA'S BERYL
                    CH. ON TIME PENNY'S CASSANDRA

232

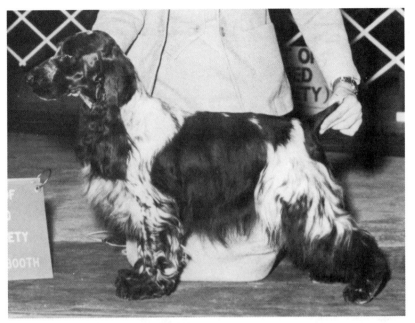

Ch. Somerset-Saga's Antigone (12/17/74).

CH. DUNELM PYGMALION
CH. DUNELM GALAXY
CH. DUNELM STARDUST
CH. KENOBO CONSTELLATION
CH. SILVER LARIOT OF STRATHPINE
CH. KENOBO MOONLIGHT MAJIC
CH. CYGNET'S RASPBERRY, CD
VARI'S INSTIGATOR
(Sire) LOCHNELL FLAMES SON OF ULWELL
CH. MAPLE LAWN TORTOISE SHELL
SEA NYMPH OF LOCHNELL
CH. VARI'S PARTY TRICKS
CH. MAPLE LAWN JAUNTI JACTATION
CH. MAPLE LAWN SLUMBER PARTY, CD
CH. MAPLE LAWN DAY DREAMER

CH. DUNELM GALAXY
CH. KENOBO CONSTELLATION
CH. KENOBO MOONLIGHT MAJIC
VARI'S WILD PARTY
CH. MAPLE LAWN JAUNTI JACTATION
CH. MAPLE LAWN SLUMBER PARTY, CD
CH. MAPLE LAWN DAY DREAMER
VARI'S PANDORA, CD
(Dam) LOCHNELL FLAMES OF ULWELL
CH. MAPLE LAWN TORTOISE SHELL
SEA NYMPH OF LOCHNELL
VARI'S BEWITCHING PARTY
CH. MAPLE LAWN JAUNTI JACTATION
CH. MAPLE LAWN SLUMBER PARTY, CD
CH. MAPLE LAWN DAY DREAMER

233

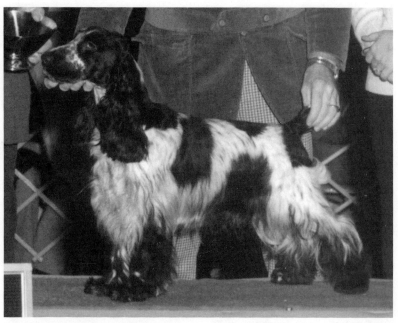

Ch. Vari's Fascination (7/2/71).   *Booth Photo*

CH. COLINWOOD BLAZE AWAY
CH. DUNELM PYGMALION
COLINWOOD WOODROYD CAROUSEL
CH. DUNELM GALAXY
CH. GLENGLADDON LUCKY STAR
CH. DUNELM STARDUST
DUNELM MERRY-GO-ROUND
CH. KENOBO CONSTELLATION
(Sire)   ENG. CH. COLINWOOD SILVER LARIOT
CH. SILVER LARIOT OF STRATHPINE
CARTREF SILVERDEW
CH. KENOBO MOONLIGHT MAJIC
CH. DUNELM HICKORY
CH. CYGNET'S RASPBERRY
SOHO BATIK

LOCHNELL FLAMES SON OF ULWELL
CH. MAPLE LAWN TORTOISE SHELL
SEA NYMPH OF LOCHNELL
CH. VARI'S PARTY TRICKS
(Dam)   CH. LOCKNELL BLUE FLASH OF ULWELL
CH. MAPLE LAWN JAUNTI JACTATION
LOCKNELL BLUE CLOUD OF ULWELL
CH. MAPLE LAWN SLUMBER PARTY, CD
MAPLE LAWN HUNTER OF HALL SAN
CH. MAPLE LAWN DAY DREAMER
CH. MERRYTHOUGH OF LOCKNELL

234

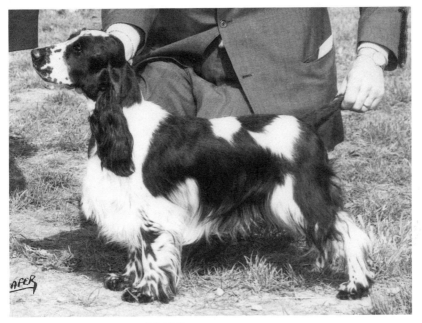

Ch. Kenobo Moonlight Majic (9/30/66). *Evelyn M. Shafer*

```
                        FANTEE SILVER SENTINEL
                   JOYWYN'S BLUE FLASH
                        CARTREF CHARMER
            ENG. CH. COLINWOOD SILVER LARIOT
                        ENG. CH. COLINWOOD FIREBRAND
                   TRUSLERS MISTY MORN
                        TRUSLER'S TRACERY
    CH. SILVER LARIOT OF STRATHPINE
         (Sire)            ENG. CH. JOYWYN'S BLUE BOY OF WARE
                   ENG. CH. DELLAH MERRYMAKER OF WYKEY
                        DELLAH MERRY MAID OF WYKEY
            CARTREF SILVERDEW
                        NOSTREBOR RIVERBANK ROGUE
                   OLICANA ISOUDE
                        OLICANA JOYBELLE


                        ENG. CH. COLINWOOD SILVER LARIOT
                   CH. COLINWOOD CHEYENNE
                        CRAIGLEITH GEISHA GIRL
            CH. DUNELM HICKORY
                        CH. JOYANNE'S DANIEL OF DUNELM
                   CH. DUNELM CHEROKEE ROSE
                        CH. DUNELM DAPHNE
    CH. CYGNET'S RASPBERRY, CD
         (Dam)            CH. SKY RIDGE ALERT
                   CH. QUARTO L. ALERT'S SON
                        STEVELYN SOLANGE
            SOHO BATIK
                        CH. ON TIME WILLIE II
                   CH. ON TIME'S OWN ANNIE
                        CH. ON TIME DEBORAH
```

Glossary

American Kennel Club (AKC)   The governing body for purebred dogs in the United States. This organization maintains stud and breeding records on all registered dogs. It also oversees dog shows, obedience trials, field trials and other sporting events and maintains records of all wins achieved under its auspices.

Angulation   The term refers to the angles created by bones meeting at various joints, especially at the shoulder, pelvis, stifle and hock.

Best of Breed   The award given to the dog or bitch who defeats all others of the same breed in competition at a given show.

Best of Opposite Sex   The award given to the best dog or bitch of the opposite sex to the one who wins Best of Breed.

Best of Winners   That dog or bitch judged best among all non-champion competitors in a given breed at AKC licensed shows.

Bitch   The female of the species.

Bite   The name given to the position of the upper and lower teeth in relation to each other when the mouth is closed. In the English Cocker the "scissors bite" is considered desirable. This occurs when the inner surfaces of the top front teeth (incisors) fit closely just over the outer surfaces of the lower front teeth. A "level bite" refers to the upper and lower teeth being lined up to meet edge to edge when the mouth is closed.

Bone Referring to substance and quality. The term "ample bone" means that the dog is sturdy and substantial in build, strong and sound, not weak or lacking in substance.

Brisket A term used to express depth of chest, which in the English Cocker should reach to the elbow.

Champion A dog or bitch who has been awarded fifteen points, including at least two wins of three or more points, at American Kennel Club licensed shows by defeating other dogs or bitches in competition.

Cobby A term referring to overall body shape, meaning that the dog should be compact in build, put together in a close-knit fashion, not long or rangy.

Companion Dog (CD) A title conferred on a dog in obedience competition that has completed certain requirements according to regulations stipulated by the American Kennel Club in licensed obedience trials. This is the basic degree awarded by AKC.

Companion Dog Excellent (CDX) This is the next degree a dog may win by completing more advanced exercises in obedience competition at AKC licensed trials.

Crate A cage made of wire, wood, fiberglass or aluminum that serves as a carrying vehicle or a safe haven for the dog either traveling or at home. Crates come in various sizes and prices, and they are extremely useful as an aid in housetraining and securing a dog at a show.

Croup The muscular area just in front of and around the set-on of the tail.

Dam Mother of the puppies.

Dog The male of the species, although often used generically to describe both males and females.

Double Coat Hair that grows dense and short next to the skin and longer and silkier on top. The hair close to the body acts as a weatherproof coat, and the top coat lies flat on the body and grows long on the belly, legs, ears and chest.

English Cocker Spaniel Club of America (ECSCA) The national club, also known as the Parent club, which is recognized by the American Kennel Club as the official organization representing the English Cocker breed and fanciers in the United States. Its functions are to promote and protect the breed, to publish a Standard of perfection for the breed, to encourage sportsmanlike competition in show, obedience and field events, and to enhance the study, breeding, exhibiting, training and maintenance of the purebred English Cocker Spaniel.

English Show Champion (Eng. Sh. Ch.)   A title earned in England that indicates that the English Cocker has won points in the show ring, but has not won a championship in the field. If a dog has won both in the field and in the show ring in England, it would be titled "champion."

Epilepsy   A neurological disorder of the brain waves of unknown origin that causes the dog to have seizures. It is a hereditary condition in English Cockers.

Ewe Neck   A neck considered an anatomical weakness because it lacks strength at the base and in which the top of the neck is concave instead of arched.

Familial Renal Disease   Also known as familial nephropathy, this is a hereditary malformation of the kidney, which affects young dogs, usually under the age of two. The dogs cannot function because the kidney does not grow properly, resulting in renal failure and death.

Field Trial Champion   A title conferred by the American Kennel Club upon a dog that shows exceptional ability in the field at licensed field trials, by winning first place in designated classes, or "stakes," a prescribed number of times, thus winning points depending upon the number of entries. Ten points are needed to become a Field Trial Champion.

Flews   The upper lips, which cover the mouth and teeth.

Gait   The way the dog moves, whether walking or trotting. It is a term used to describe movement in the show ring.

Get   Offspring or produce of the sire.

Grain of the Hair   The direction in which the hair grows. Clipping with the grain means running the clippers in the same direction in which the hair grows. Clipping against the grain means clipping in the direction opposite to which the hair grows.

Grooming   Brushing, combing and general maintenance of the dog, including cleaning teeth, clipping nails and bathing.

Hare Foot   A foot on which the middle toes are elongated, like a rabbit. This is a fault in English Cockers.

Haws   The rims or margins of the lower eyelids. When the lower lids are loose, they expose the inner lining of the lids, causing a condition that promotes irritation and infection.

Hip Dysplasia   A hereditary condition in which there is abnormal laxity in the hip joints, causing arthritic changes leading to lameness.

Hock   A joint on the rear leg connecting the lower thigh and the rear pastern. Often the hock is used to describe the bone connecting the lower thigh to the rear foot.

Junior Hunter   A title awarded to a dog that has completed a variety of tests in the field to ascertain hunting ability. These tests are sponsored by the American Kennel Club.

Loin   The area of the body extending from the end of the rib cage to the start of the pelvis.

Master Hunter   The highest AKC title a dog can achieve in a series of tests to determine its ability in the field. The hunting tests are not competitive, whereas AKC licensed field trials are competitive with the awarding of placements. Hunting tests are pass/fail tests for each dog.

Mismark   Colors or patterns in the coat that are not allowed in the Standard for the breed—in English Cockers, for instance, white feet on an all black dog.

Nail Clipper   A tool used to cut the ends of the toenails. There are basically two types, the guillotine type, in which the nail is placed into a round opening in the clipper, and the pincher type, which operates like a garden tool.

Obedience Trial Champion (OTCH)   The highest title a dog can achieve in obedience competition. It must win a total of 100 points in AKC licensed obedience trials to qualify for this title.

Occiput   The point at the rear of the skull that is important in defining the correct head. Anatomically it serves as a location for the attachment of muscles of the head and the back of the neck. It is the peak of the back skull.

Overshot A receding lower jaw that causes the upper front teeth to protrude too far over the lower front teeth, so there is no contact between them.

Progeny The offspring of either the sire or the dam, or both.

Progressive Retinal Atrophy (PRA) This is a hereditary disease in which the retina of the eye gradually disintegrates, causing blindness. It is carried by a recessive gene, meaning that both sire and dam must be carriers in order for the offspring to become blind. Breeders who have a blind dog do not use it for breeding, and do not use either of the parents. In English Cockers PRA does not manifest itself until the dog is three or four years old.

Prosternum The portion of the breastbone, sometimes called forechest, that projects beyond the point at which the shoulder meets the upper arm.

Quick That portion of the toenail which contains blood vessels and nerves.

Roan A color pattern created by a mixture of colored and white hairs. Roaning is distinct from color patches because of the white, which is evenly mixed in. Blue roan is a mixture of black and white. Roan patterns are also seen in orange, lemon and liver colors.

Scale of Points The schedule promulgated by the American Kennel Club to determine the number in competition required for championship points in each breed at AKC licensed shows throughout the United States. The requirements for points vary with regions of the country. The largest number of points a dog can win at any one show is five. The smallest is one.

Senior Hunter An AKC title conferred upon a dog that completes certain tests to determine its ability in the field. It is the second level of achievement, the first being Junior Hunter, the top being Master Hunter.

Shelly A term describing a dog who lacks substance and gives the appearance of lacking strength and sufficient muscle and bone mass.

Short-coupled The description used for a dog when the distance between the last rib and the beginning of the hindquarters is relatively short. A short-coupled dog is usually considered to be strong through the back and loins.

Sire   The father of the puppies.

Special   A term given to a champion who is competing for Best of Breed competition.

Specialty   A dog show that is limited to one breed, as distinct from an all-breed show, in which all breeds licensed by the American Kennel Club may compete.

Splay Foot   A foot that is flat where the toes are spread, causing weakness in the foot.

Standard   A description of the breed that was developed by the fanciers of that breed, usually through the actions of a club. The Standard describes the ideal appearance and character of the breed and is the model toward which breeders strive. Dog show judges use the Standard to attempt to find the dogs that most closely fit the description in awarding ribbons and championship points.

Stifle   The joint in the hind leg that connects the upper and lower thigh. The degree of angle formed at this juncture determines the angulation of the hindquarter.

Stripping   The procedure of pulling out undercoat on the body, head and sides using a stripping knife or stone.

Substance   The description used to indicate whether a dog has sufficient bone and body mass to appear sturdy and strong.

Ticked   A description of a basically white dog that has flecks of color throughout the hair. A ticked coat has less color than roan throughout.

Topline   The back from shoulders to croup is considered to be the topline. The Standard describes the topline for the English Cocker as being short and strong without dip or sagginess.

Tracking Dog (TD)   An AKC obedience title conferred on a dog that completes tests to determine its ability to follow a scent that has been laid down along a prescribed course.

Tracking Dog Excellent (TDX)   An advanced AKC degree conferred on a dog that completes more difficult tests to determine its ability to follow a scent.

Trimming   The procedure of clipping, scissoring and stripping the coat to achieve the desired appearance, usually for the show ring.

Tuck-up   The contour of the underline, or abdomen, from the chest to the beginning of the hindquarters.

Undershot   A description of the mouth in which the lower jaw protrudes beyond the upper jaw, causing the lower front teeth to grow in front of the upper front teeth.

Utility Dog (UD)   An advanced AKC title in obedience competition in which the dog performs certain exercises to determine its ability to follow commands. It is the most difficult level a dog can achieve, and follows the CDX title.

Whelp   To give birth to a litter. A whelp is a newborn puppy.

Winners   The award given to a non-champion dog and bitch in each breed at a show to designate that dog as the one winning the points awarded at that show. Winners Dog and Winners Bitch then compete for the award of Best of Winners.

Withers   The area at the junction of the base of the neck and the back at which the shoulder blades are joined to the spine. It is the highest point of the back and is the place where the back begins.

Working Dog (WD)   A title conferred by the breed club—in English Cockers, the English Cocker Spaniel Club of America—on a dog that performs certain tests to determine its hunting ability.

Working Dog Excellent (WDX)   An advanced title conferred by the English Cocker Spaniel Club of America on a dog that satisfactorily performs tests in addition to the working dog tests to determine its hunting ability.